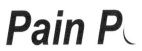

# Pain Prophecies

## *Finding Meaning in the Fire*

## Girl God Books

Edited by Kay Louise Aldred,
Pat Daly, and Trista Hendren

Cover Art by Kat Shaw

©2023 All Rights Reserved
ISBN: 978-82-93725-49-7

**www.thegirlgod.com**

# Praise for Pain Perspectives

"When first approached to write an endorsement for this book I felt quietly confident. I have been a practitioner of Classical Chinese medicine and somatic therapies for forty years, and pain is my compassion language. I know pain in all its forms both professionally and personally. So, all good, right?

But the collection of essays, poems and art in this anthology is so visceral and on point that there was nothing easy about the read or the analysis. Chronic pain, institutionalized pain, cultural pain, all washing over us mentally, physically, and spiritually. All is beautifully explored and poignantly written here.

And while we are neurologically wired to retract from pain, I do believe we need to feel it, name it, and stare it down in order to move past it. This important anthology will help us all to do that. Read it and cherish the awakened sensations as you would with your tongue playing with a loose tooth. And then we get up tomorrow and do what needs to be done."

-Gina Martin, author of the *When She Wakes* series (*Sisters of the Solstice Moon, Walking the Threads of Time, She is Here*),  the *Daughters of the Goddess* series (*Kiyia-Daughter of the Horse*), and *WomEnchanting*, a compendium of sacred songs and chants


"Once again, Girl God books – and the courageous women who share that has been banished to the shadows, silenced, disparaged, and demonized – is a profoundly valuable gift to everyone who is being called to reintegrate our feminine receptive nature.

*Pain Perspectives* is a beautiful sharing of how the pain of existing in a heart-and-soul deprived patriarchal paradigm has been endured – and has contributed to women's wisdom, gifts, and soul's evolution. A must read for anyone who has lived with pain, whether physical, emotional, or spiritual. Pretty much everyone. The women who traveled to the depths, transmuted their pain, garnered the wisdom, and rose to inspire others is an authentic depiction of the energy of the Goddess returning through each and every one of us. I recommend taking your time to receive each story in this book, as deeply as it was shared."

-Mary Lane, author of *Divine Nourishment & Meena*

# Girl God Books

### The Crone Initiation: Women Speak on the Menopause Journey

*The Crone Initiation* is an anthology of women's experiences of perimenopause and menopause, and the part Goddess plays in this journey. Crone's presence in the breakdowns and breakthroughs, the disintegration and rebuilding, is expressed through words and art. Meaning is reclaimed and the power of the Elder restored.

### Re-Membering with Goddess: Healing the Patriarchal Perpetuation of Trauma

*Re-Membering with Goddess* is an anthology of women's experiences of trauma—trauma as a result of patriarchy; trauma perpetuated by patriarchy; and how through personal healing of trauma the Goddess is re-membered, re-embodied and resurrected. As repeating loops of trauma restriction release—in the mind, body and nervous system—Goddess is re-embodied and rises... and the patriarchy falls.

### Just as I Am: Hymns Affirming the Divine Female

*What is a Hermnal?* It's the collective sigh of our ancestral Grandmothers. It's a means of drawing us closer together as Sisters. It is a compilation of songs that affirm our Sacredness, apart from Man, and assures us that we are Sovereign Beings and Creatrixes, too. And it is our Love Gift of Gratitude to Mama.

### Songs of Solstice: Goddess Carols

This Songbook celebrates the cycles of Nature—Birth, Life, and Death—through the changing Seasons (the Turning of the Wheel) from Autumn's abundance, for which we give thanks, to Winter's "Dead Time," when even the warmth of the Sun leaves us, and the world goes dark and cold. It is a celebration of both the Light and the Dark, since both are Sacred and both are needed for new Life to grow and flourish.

### The Girl God

A book for children young and old, celebrating the Divine Female by Trista Hendren. Magically illustrated by Elisabeth Slettnes with quotes from various faith traditions and feminist thinkers.

### Re-visioning Medusa: from Monster to Divine Wisdom

A remarkable collection of essays, poems, and art by scholars who have researched Her, artists who have envisioned Her, and women who have known Her in their personal story. All have spoken with Her and share something of their communion in this anthology.

### In Defiance of Oppression – The Legacy of Boudicca

An anthology that encapsulates the Spirit of the defiant warrior in a modern apathetic age. No longer will the voices of our sisters go unheard, as the ancient Goddesses return to the battlements, calling to ignite the spark within each and every one of us—to defy oppression wherever we find it, and stand together in solidarity.

### Warrior Queen: Answering the Call of The Morrigan

A powerful anthology about the Irish Celtic Goddess. Each contributor brings The Morrigan to life with unique stories that invite readers to partake and inspire them to pen their own. Included are essays, poems, stories, chants, rituals, and art from dozens of storytellers and artists from around the world, illustrating and recounting the many ways this powerful Goddess of war, death, and prophecy has changed their lives.

### Inanna's Ascent: Reclaiming Female Power

Inanna's Ascent examines how females can rise from the underworld and reclaim their power, sovereignly expressed through poetry, prose and visual art. All contributors are extraordinary women in their own right, who have been through some difficult life lessons—and are brave enough to share their stories.

### Willendorf's Legacy: The Sacred Body

Travel through time and discover a world where the fullness of women was both admired and deified. Reclaim your beautiful Goddess body through the rich pages of this powerful collection of art, poetry and essays celebrating our divine inheritance as daughters of Willendorf.

**Complete list of Girl God publications at www.thegirlgod.com**

"True resistance begins with people confronting pain...
and wanting to do something to change it."

-bell hooks

## *Dedication:*

For the liberation of all women's bodies.

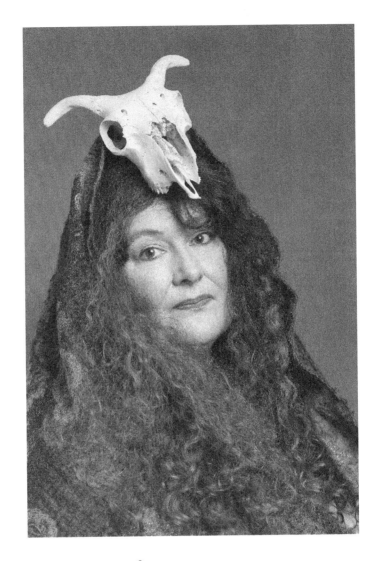

**In remembrance** of our beloved sister
and fellow contributor Barbara O'Meara.

(April 11th, 1963 – October 5th, 2023)

Rest in Power and in Peace.

We love you Barbara.

Photo by Marta Faye Photography, "The Veil is Thin." 2020.

# Table of Contents

# Pain Perspectives:
## This is my Body. Broken with You.

### Kay Louise Aldred

Day-to-day I live with, and manage, chronic pain – alongside millions of other women.

Globally it is estimated that 30% of the world population experiences chronic pain. I'm one of them. This is my body. This type of pain affects more women than men. I'm one of them. Broken with you.

The reason I decided on this particular title for this article – which is a play on eucharistic and biblical phrase "Take, eat; this is my body which is given for you; do this in remembrance of me" – is because those of us who were raised in the Christian tradition will have heard a variation of these words and no doubt have pondered what they actually mean – within worship, bible study and religious education classes. Inevitably, through these words we have been 'programmed', to some extent, that the body is to be 'given away' or 'sacrificed' to intense suffering, for the sake of and to 'feed' 'another' and/or 'God', and that pain and suffering are an acceptable exchange, in God's view, for redemption. This 'programme' layers on top of other Christian conditioning we have received around the body being sinful and 'base'.

**Pain Perspective – This is my body**

The human body is not meant to live in a state of perpetual pain. The reasons for chronic pain, according to medical professionals, are complex and often unexplainable. Whilst I may experience pain in my body it is not a case for me that 'this is my body' – the pain is not my body – it doesn't define it. It is an aspect of what I process within it. In simultaneously meditating on the words 'this is my body' and feeling pain within it – I have observed the body and the pain are two distinct and separate things.

Shamanic journeying has given me significant insight into the origins of the pain I feel. Much of it is a physical manifestation of unresolved ancestral patterning and trauma. This is not 'my' body. It is the ancestral trauma body. The majority of it is patriarchal, societal and religious conditioning – lack of rest, overworking, lack of pleasure. The pain is an objection to this. It seems my body has been 'given away' to intense suffering for the sake of the continuation of the patriarchy and has been a resource for a man (to raise his children), the state (as an unpaid carer of my parents and children) and the education system (as a teacher). My body's pain and suffering keep male omnipotence, a 'Big Daddy' rulership, in place and I am, according to the Christian narrative, redeemed and favoured because of my self-sacrifice. The Christian story and dynamic continue to play out, interestingly, I notice, and primarily within and through the female body. The male body has even been able to shirk that responsibility. I wonder what the stories and perspectives of other women are about pain and their body and their understanding of the link.

**Pain Perspective – Broken with You**

Whilst in the Eucharist, the bread is broken. For this article I wanted to explore the concept of 'broken body' and how it relates to pain. When I looked up the definition of the word broken, I saw a range of words which did not resonate with my experience of pain. Of the non-resonant words, three especially did not fit my personal experience of pain – these words were 'imperfect', 'not functioning' and 'severely damaged'. Pain is not an imperfection from my perspective. Pain is a perfect sensation – absolute, complete, having all the qualities for its function – alerting me to a message from my body; that it needs extra care or attention. Pain also demonstrates that my body is functioning effectively and is undamaged and actually fulfilling its task of sending a message.

The resonant definitions of the word broken in relation to my perspective of pain were 'interrupted' and 'fractured'. The pain I experience interrupts my sleepwalking through life and unconsciously perpetuating and participating in the patriarchal play I am a character in and acting out. The pain stops me in my tracks. What I have observed is that the onset of pain happens when I am too much 'in my head', serving others without reciprocation and/or neglecting my pleasure. So, from that viewpoint, the pain is an ally, showing me that I am imbalanced, fractured from joy, embodiment, Goddess and the feminine. And as the words say broken with you – they remind me that I am not alone in feeling this. My body, along with the bodies of millions of other Sisters are discerning through sensation that how we are living is not in alignment with health, spirit or joy and we are rejecting the old patriarchal patterning.

My intuition is that the worldwide epidemic of chronic pain is an inflammatory response in humanity to the invasion of patriarchy and its effects. Our collective spiritual and physical immune system is reacting and saying NO. The wisdom of pain is showing us we are out of alignment with our natural, embodied, human birthright – pleasure, wellness and ease.

Pain is a political and revolutionary statement from the body. A clear message that society, paradigms, culture and systems – and religious narrative – need to change.

# *Surviving*

## Barbara O'Meara

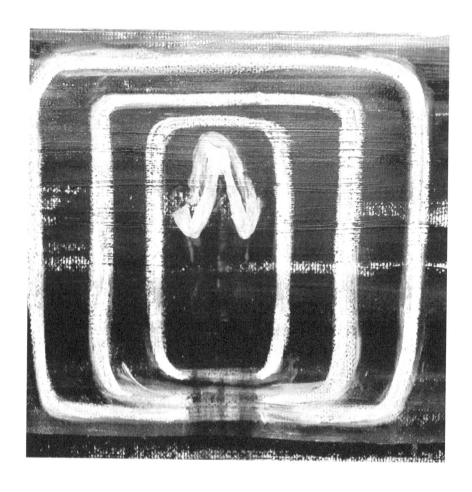

# *Styles and Preferences*

Trista Hendren

*Pain Perspectives* contains a variety of writing styles from people around the world. Various forms of English are included in this anthology and we chose to keep spellings of the writers' place of origin to honor/honour each individual's unique voice.

It was the expressed intent of the editors to not police standards of citation, transliteration and formatting. Contributors have determined which citation style, italicization policy and transliteration system to adopt in their pieces. The resulting diversity is a reflection of the diversity of academic fields, genres and personal expressions represented by the authors.[1]

Mary Daly wrote long ago that, "Women have had the power of naming stolen from us."[2] The quest for our own naming, and our own language, is never-ending, and each of us attempts it differently.

People often get caught up on whether we say Goddess or *Girl God* or *Divine Female* vs. *Divine Feminine*. Personally, I try to just listen to what the speaker is trying to say. The fact remains that few of us were privileged with a woman-affirming education—and we all have a lot of time to make up for. Let's all be gentle with each other through that process.

If you find that a particular writing doesn't sit well with you, please feel free to use the Al-Anon suggestion: "Take what you like, leave the rest!" That said, if there aren't at least several pieces that challenge you, we have not done our job here.

---

[1] This paragraph is borrowed and adapted with love from *A Jihad for Justice: Honoring the Work and Life of Amina Wadud*. Edited by Kecia Ali, Juliane Hammer and Laury Silvers.

[2] Daly, Mary. *Gyn/Ecology: The Metaethics of Radical Feminism*. Beacon Press, 1990.

# Do Chronic Pain and Illness Have Inherent Meaning?

### Sylvia Rose

Cultural attitudes toward disability, chronic illness (both physical and mental), pain and sensory impairments are strikingly varied across time and place. All sorts of meanings have been projected onto disability: some positive, some not, some now unknowable to us.

In parts of ancient Greece, babies born visibly imperfect were exposed on hillsides and left to die. Yet by contrast, excavations of bodies from ancient settlements in the Orkneys reveal skeletons of adults with clear disabilities, including blindness and arthritis. Such people would have struggled to take care of themselves in a hostile agrarian landscape, so in order to reach adulthood and beyond their families and friends must have cared for them, fed them from their limited supplies of food, and valued them. Were they perhaps the ones who stayed home by the fire, who had time to think, to dream, to talk to the Goddess? Were their disabilities seen as making them somehow more sacred?

In Siberian Shamanic tradition it was often the experience of misfortune, including prolonged illness, that brought people into their power. It was the upheaval of daily life, the break in ordinary routines, the dislocation, the empty time for communing with the spirits – for seeing and truly knowing what matters most – that led them to the path of becoming a shaman.

And sometimes in myths, disability was the necessary trade that Gods and heroes made for coming into their full power. Odin gained his wisdom in his nine nights upon the tree, but he gave an eye in return. Sedna lost her fingers and was unable to care for herself, but the sea creatures loved her and took care of her. Sacrifice brings its rewards. Disability brings gain.

How many contemporary notions have now moved away from these ideas? Now, people with chronic illness or pain are more often the object of charity, are seen as expensive and not necessarily deserving recipients of welfare state largesse. Occasional physical achievements are lauded with a tinge of pity or condescension: Look, he has no arms or legs, but he still managed to run from Land's End to John O'Groats. Whereas in truth, living with a chronic impairment makes you neither a hero nor a tragic figure – just someone for whom life has taken a different, more complex and challenging path.

So people can forget to ask what spiritual gifts people on these paths can bring to their community. How someone with sight difficulties can teach us to tune into the natural world with other senses. How the need to develop self-healing practices teaches sensitivity to energy working of all kinds. How priorities look different for someone in bed all day, someone differently-abled.

If anything, the rhetoric of our society is that illnesses are sent to teach us some lesson. Which brings the unfortunate corollary that if we're still ill, it's because we haven't quite understood the reason yet. That if we die, it's because we got something wrong. That the Goddess or the Universe doesn't love us quite enough to heal us, or we haven't said our prayers to her quite right, haven't evolved far enough down our spiritual path, haven't hugged enough trees yet. This is a nice exercise in denial, but untrue; springing more probably from an unacknowledged fear of illness and death happening to us ourselves. Illusions of control. There must be something you can do about it all. Don't let it beat you.

And maybe some lingering animal herd instinct, to shun those who can't keep up with the rest, who are visibly suffering or weak. And the frustrations and deep scariness of caring deeply for someone whose daily pain and illness you are powerless to help. We all hate powerlessness: It's easier to suppress it and blame the person themself for not recovering faster. "I'm sure you would feel better if only you..." How many times have I heard that?

In truth, illness comes equally to those who are a long way down their spiritual path and those who aren't. And what meaning it might have gone far deeper than the question of can we make ourselves well again. These matters are not for anyone else to judge, to impose their own meanings on. These meanings are ours alone to seek.

Despite the teachings of our contemporary capitalist society, your worth is not measured by your productivity. Your value to your ritual group is not measured by how far you can climb uphill. Let's celebrate differences and look for what we can all learn from each other.

## *Silenced*
Kat Shaw

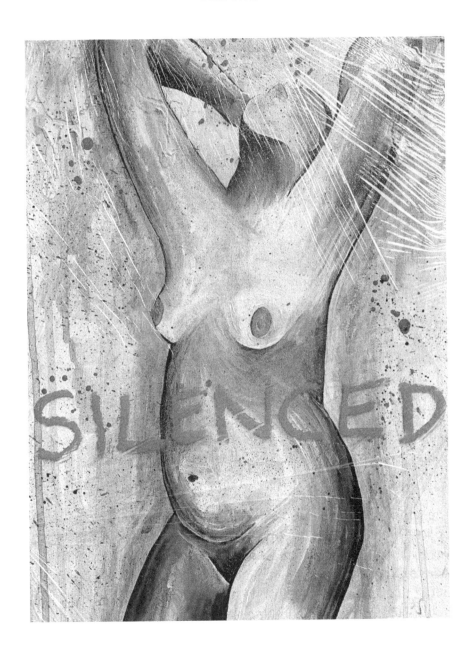

# Rebirthing Through the Underworld Goddesses

Alison Newvine

My journey with chronic pain began as a whisper. Like the scratch of a fly's legs along the side of my neck, the discomfort persisted with occasional jabs of a hotter, fiercer sting. The roots of the pain go back further to that vulnerable time when children learn to inhabit fragile bodies that discharge shockwaves of overwhelming physical sensation in response to shame, fear, anger and other emotional throes.

The foundations for chronic pain were in place by the time I moved to the Bay Area, California at age twenty-four. As a highly sensitive queer kid in a small, conservative, Christian town, I saw problems others didn't see and felt harm that seemed imperceptible to everyone else. My mother held infinite space for my distress and the chaos my sensitivity appeared to be causing in our family. Yet, try as she might, she couldn't really understand me. We were both hopelessly confused and she had her own chronic illness brewing.

I believe the point of origin for her pain and mine go back further than either of us can remember. Generation upon generation of sensitive beings severed from life affirming, embodied spirituality and covered in a shroud of patriarchal religion offering no warmth, no comfort, only suffocation.

The father god teaches us to override what's going on in our bodies, in the temples of our creativity and our wisdom. Stand, sit, kneel. Don't think, don't question, don't feel. Original thought is akin to Original Sin and the feminine is, at best, inferior. I broke out of the choking confines of the Catholic faith at age fourteen, but the mechanisms of numbing and tensing against the onslaught of psychic sensation and emotion remained deeply rooted. The splitting apart of shadow and radiance, and the accompanying shame and helplessness were wired in my brain, body and dreamworld. For now, there was no escape.

Years living in the Bay Area slowly transformed my defiant atheism into an agnosticism with pagan leanings. The Goddess wasn't difficult to find in this corner of the world. I found her in a dozen bookstores, old record albums, chance conversations, images on postcards and other people's tattoos. She started as a mystery, a longing, a fantasy that hinted at something like a memory. In time, She came closer.

As I began to reweave some threads of connection between body and mind through practicing yoga and working with a body-oriented psychotherapist, the Goddess just showed up. I began to drum and sing the Earth Goddess chants I'd been hearing. I found community centering around the Sacred Feminine and my creativity blossomed. The Muse had awakened. I began writing my own music in praise of the Divine Mother and in sorrow and protest of the damaging impact of patriarchy and religious oppression. I became a yoga teacher, enrolled in a graduate program in psychology and was mapping out a future that felt aligned.

Oddly, the closer I came to the Goddess, the more intense the pain became. Perhaps that is one of the ways She came to be feared in the first place. Goddess is Life, and living comes with pain. Coming to know the Goddess in her many forms quickened in me the impulse to self-actualize, to shed what isn't me and synchronize more fully with my Soul. This is not a painless path.

Even in the modern Goddess consciousness practices and communities, an imprint of patriarchal religion lives on. In our desire to end suffering, we reach for the luminous and push anything that doesn't scream "love and light" into the shadows. We disown parts of our psyche that are not inherently bad, but can become toxic when shut away in the closet. What we lack in the shadow realm, we unconsciously project onto others, creating disharmony in our relationships and communities. For those of us socialized female, the mandate to be nice leads us to sacrifice our needs and override our own healthy boundaries. Relationships become unsustainable. Health deteriorates. Continuously overriding our needs, feelings and boundaries often show up as physical pain in our bodies. The body *is* the shadow realm.

From my very early Goddess days, I was captivated by the story of Ereshkigal and Inanna. Dwelling in the light above, Inanna descends into the underworld to meet her sister, Ereshkigal, who resides in the shadows below. Ereshkigal forces Inanna to strip away layers of her protective persona, represented by losing a garment at each of the seven gates of the underworld. Ereshkigal's role is to confront Inanna with her own shadow, including the impact of her unconscious actions. It is a story about integrating the shadow into the conscious personality, and the painful shedding of identity and ego death that is required for this integration to take place.

By the end of 2019, my physical pain was reaching new levels. Until that point the pain had been localized in my back and neck and now I was experiencing tingling, sharp pains in my hands that began interfering with activities of daily living. I was a newly licensed therapist with a caseload building faster than my body and psyche could keep up with. The year 2019 was the beginning of a descent into a collective and personal underworld. That year closed with an intentional yet rushed and chaotic upheaval of foundational structures of my life that I believed would be quickly rebuilt once my partner and I were settled in our new home in early 2020.

My nervous system had been stressed beyond capacity for an extended period of time when, in early 2020, COVID-19 changed all of our lives. I entered this era with an empty tank and a broken body. I'll admit, initially I was relieved to have a break from the outside world. Social relating had been feeling overwhelming and there was an impulse toward isolation that the external circumstances were now contriving to support. The glamor of shadow projection had fooled me into thinking that if I could just get away from people, I would feel peace.

The pandemic awakened in many of us unconscious memories of early childhood and preverbal trauma. Fear, uncertainty and helplessness evoked these bodily memories. I saw it in my psychotherapy practice, in my home, in myself. For those of us quarantining with partners, the shadow projection within the couple relationship amped up in the absence of other relationships to share this burden. I saw this in countless couples I worked with in my practice during this time and my spouse and I were no exception to this phenomenon.

We were all being forced to undertake Inanna's journey to meet Ereshkigal. The more I resisted, the more my body became a prison. The physical pain progressed alongside the psychological distress and mounting feelings of helplessness. Eventually, I lost the ability to go for walks, play the guitar, write in my journal and even feed myself without assistance due to the unbearable pain. Panic attacks and insomnia accompanied the physical pain and loss of mobility. There was no escape. I felt forsaken.

But I wasn't alone, not really. Hekate, Goddess of the Crossroads was there with her torch and her powerful magic presiding over me as I slowly transformed in this underworld. She worked with me in those painful hours, nights, months. Her presence wasn't as all-consuming as I longed for and there were many times I couldn't feel Her at all, nor could I remember to call out for Her. She was both there and not there. She wasn't going to do the work for me. She was going to give me just enough help so that I could chose to walk Inanna's path myself and shed the worn-out garments that were painfully stuck to my skin.

Isolation taught me that every agonizing thing I experience *out there* is also *in here.* I had to see and reclaim the shadows I had projected onto others. I had to meet my Ereshkigal and, through compassion, restore her to her original essence, unite with her. I had to tend to the little girl suddenly awake and terrified within me. I had to feel my anger and start honoring my physical, emotional and psychic boundaries. I had to feel the desire to die and allow myself to see what was truly ready to die in me before I could be reborn. I had to **become** the Underworld Goddess, guiding myself through the hell that collective/personal trauma and poisonous defensive structures had created.

In time, I came to understand that the intensity of the physical pain correlated to the fear and resistance I was feeling. This understanding broke open an underground wellspring of magical tools to transform my experience of physical pain. Hekate's keys were becoming mine. The underworld journey showed me that the splitting apart of my shadow and my radiance breeds fear and pain. The key is to accept it all, unconditionally, over and over again. It isn't a revelation, it is a practice. That early programming of God above and devil below, an afterlife of eternal bliss or endless torture is a perversion of reality. The bliss and the torture are here, within and around each of us. The heaven/hell construct teaches that pain is to be feared and motivation toward good comes from trying to avoid the fires of hell.

The fires of the Goddess are completely different.

She transforms us through Her fires. She doesn't keep us there for all eternity because we have made mistakes, harmed others or failed to go to church every Sunday. She teaches that the underworld is *indwelling* and Goddess walks with us there as much as She walks with us in the light. She is the light in the dark and the dark in the light.

An unexpected guide in my ongoing journey with chronic pain has been Cerridwen, a being who exists between worlds. In her story, she chases after an initiate who took her magic wisdom potion. He changes into various animal forms trying to elude her and she changes forms to pursue him until he becomes a grain of wheat and she consumes him. He transmogrifies within her belly and is rebirthed into his next incarnation as singer and storyteller, the wisdom he sought now assimilated into his being. Cerridwen teaches that a glorious transformation awaits if we let go. We fear punishment, we fear dissolution. But the energy of the Goddess is inherently loving. There is no eternal hellfire. Only eternal change.

Accepting my shadow means accepting not only chronic pain but the anger and anxiety I feel in response to it. The more of myself that I accept, the less the pain controls me. It still roars and rages and burns. But I no longer fear it or feel punished by it. I go for beautiful walks in nature, I'm cooking, building community, playing my guitar. And sometimes I just rest. I've begun writing songs in praise of the Goddesses of the Underworld. Cerridwen's symbolism is also that of Muse, inspiring centuries of songs arising from that moment of dissolution and regeneration.

I understand what causes and exacerbates the pain more now than I ever have. Yet, its persistence humbles me. There's still so much more about it that I *don't* understand and have not resolved. The presence of chronic pain challenges me to see and care for myself in new and evolving ways. Healthy, unapologetic boundaries and fierce shadow work are at the center of my ongoing healing as are the Underworld Goddesses- Ereshkigal, Inanna, Hekate, Cerridwen. Do I wish I could live each day, or even one day, without the presence of pain? Of course. Do I accept and embrace that a painless path is not what I am walking? Also, yes. I feel more myself now than before the descent and rebirthing. I have committed to seeing my chronic pain as a lifelong invitation into the Mystery. The Underworld Goddesses have so much more to teach me.

# *Devil Woman*
Rachael Noton

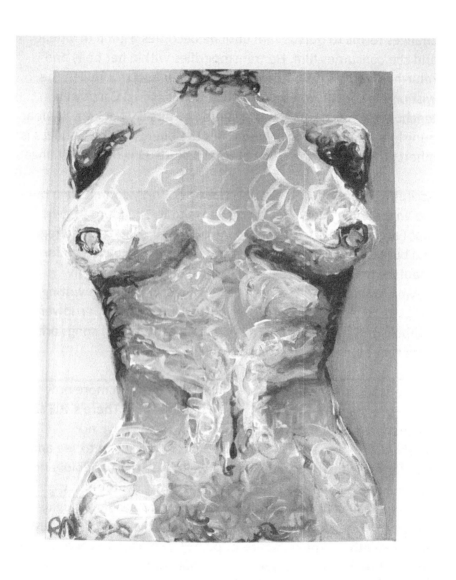

# *Pain*

### Lucy H. Pearce

Pain steals in unseen
And takes
My body, my energy, my mind.
My future, my certainty, my past.
My trust, my voice, my hope.
Pain leaves me writhing
Hostage to its demands.
I must reclaim each facet of myself from its hands,
Take a stand for this self that I never was too sure about
For this body, this mind, this life.
To claim them as my own.
At last,
The prize I always had but never truly wanted
Becomes the thing I will die trying to reclaim
From the grasping hands of pain.
This life which time and again I have
Dismissed, despaired of, overlooked, bemoaned.
*Will you fight for it now?* pain asks.

# *Pain*
Kat Shaw

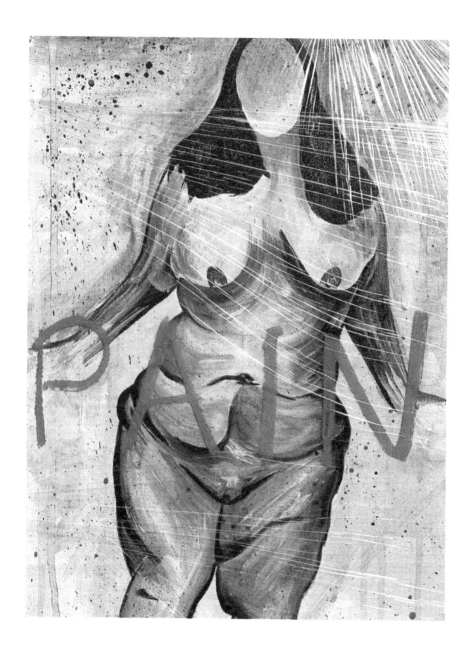

# *Pain/Killing*

Lucy H. Pearce

We are addicted to the magic trick of conjuring away pain.

We have been silencing pain for generations. The pain of wars, massacres, abuses, immigrations, famines, illness, childbirth... We are individually, collectively trying to hush the waves of darkness that keep crashing and crashing belatedly on the shores of our bodyminds. Trying to keep it down, keep it in, get back to normal. The drugs may work for a week or a month, but the waves breach their barrier and we increase our dose. Keep the waters back, the feelings down, the tears in. Nobody wants to hear it, nobody wants to see it. We just don't have the time. We don't have the energy. There is nowhere safe to collapse. We must carry on. And on. And on.

Patriarchal medicine entered into a war on pain and the terms were clear: Either we kill it, or it kills us. And they believed that they were winning the war, that we could eradicate pain forever. But our cultural reliance on magic bullets is backfiring. Rather than eliminating our pain, these bullets are taking our lives. What seemed like the easy option, of opiate painkillers to treat people with back problems, after car accidents and surgery has started an epidemic of opioid addiction. Instead of being the magic answer, painkillers have morphed into the most dangerous public health epidemic of the modern age. We are seeing how false the cultural barrier between legal and illegal drugs is.

We see a strange double standard: Running a ruthless war on "illegal" drugs at the same time that more humans than ever in the history of the planet are reliant on psychotropic medicines prescribed by doctors, many of which are of questionable efficacy. And yet some of the so-called illegal drugs (such as MDMA, LSD and marijuana), which are known to be of use in therapeutic settings where there are few effective treatments available, are banned. We have a deep cultural distrust of changing consciousness – and yet every day millions of people have their consciousness legally altered with general anaesthetics and opioid painkillers like codeine and morphine, with alcohol and even screens. We are against people choosing to use mind altering substances for personal use, to change their experience of reality, to heal, but are all too happy to prescribe them to ensure people remain functional in this dysfunctional reality when it suits us.

According to the most recent National Survey of Drug Use and Health just shy of 100 million Americans used, or misused, prescription pain pills in 2015.[3] That's almost 30% of the entire population, with 80% of people getting hooked on (supposedly non-addictive) opioids after being prescribed them. Described by the US National Institute on Drug Abuse as "a serious national crisis", opioid addictions cost US communities 100 lives a day and $78.5 billion a year.[4]

This escalation in use is not inevitable. Nor is it bad luck. Government, pharmaceutical companies and doctors are complicit in it. According to a special report by *The Guardian* newspaper, "Pharmaceutical companies spend far more than any other industry to influence politicians. Drugmakers have poured close to $2.5bn into lobbying and funding members of Congress over the past decade."[5] A former head of the Drug Enforcement Agency told the Washington Post, "The drug industry, the manufacturers, wholesalers, distributors and chain drugstores,

---

[3]www.samhsa.gov/data/sites/default/files/NSDUH-FFR1-2015/NSDUH-FFR1-2015/NSDUH-FFR1-2015.pdf
[4]www.drugabuse.gov/drugs-abuse/opioids/opioid-crisis
[5]www.theguardian.com/us-news/2017/oct/19/big-pharma-money-lobbying-us-opioid-crisis

have an influence over Congress that has never been seen before."[6]

It is no coincidence either that the type of medication people are becoming addicted to – opioids – "bind to the areas of the brain that control pain and emotions, driving up the levels of the feel-good hormone dopamine."[7] They are drugs that kill not only the physical pain that people are suffering, but also the harrowing emotional pain of living in a dying culture. And we are *all* ingesting these medications, whether or not we are prescribed them, as most urban water and seafood is now laced with excreted traces of opioids, anti-depressants and the contraceptive pill.[8]

We feel so much pain. Inside, outside. And our culture is not good at dealing with pain. It likes to bury it, numb it, hide it, ignore it. It likes having the ability to carry pain away on one simple pill and have to think no more about it. It prefers to leave aside the messiness of where it came from and why, where it's leading to and how.

Like a thousand fire alarms going off through the night, pain wails as we run in this direction and that, trying to put out the fires. We have been running so long, through the chaos, the smoke, the overwhelm and the adrenaline, our nervous systems are exhausted. But still the alarms are ringing. We long for an end to the suffering. We watch the clock, creeping forward, each second, each minute and still the pain remains… we look ahead to endless deserts barren of joy, populated only by pain. When will it end? It feels like it will outlast us. We sacrifice more and more of our body, our life, to assuaging the pain, to keeping it at bay. We grow

---

[6]www.washingtonpost.com/graphics/2017/investigations/dea-drug-industry-congress/?utm_term=.3ecbea861420
[7]edition.cnn.com/2017/09/18/health/opioid-crisis-fast-facts/index.html
[8]www.theguardian.com/us-news/2018/may/26/traces-of-opioids-found-in-mussels-in-seattle-bay

desperate and agitated in the face of its permanence, our concentration, joy, mobility, sociability, identities gradually erased by the pain, until we are living in an invisible circle – just us... and the pain... and its cousins, misery, despair and exhaustion. We lose ourselves to it. Powerless in its grasp.

In our culture we try to separate our physical pain from emotional pain and declare them to be two separate territories. Each of us has a different pain we carry, in different places in our bodies and souls. We have so much pain, that we can no long bear to feel it. We feel so much pain that we are too scared or ashamed to name it. In the abyss we find it hard to know what is my pain, what is your pain, what is our collective pain, what is old pain and what is new, and what can be done about any of it.

We can't take it anymore. It all just hurts.
We are done with it.

And so we swallow down what they offer, hoping to find relief, at last.

(From *Medicine Woman: reclaiming the soul of healing* – Lucy H. Pearce)

# *Invisible*

## Kat Shaw

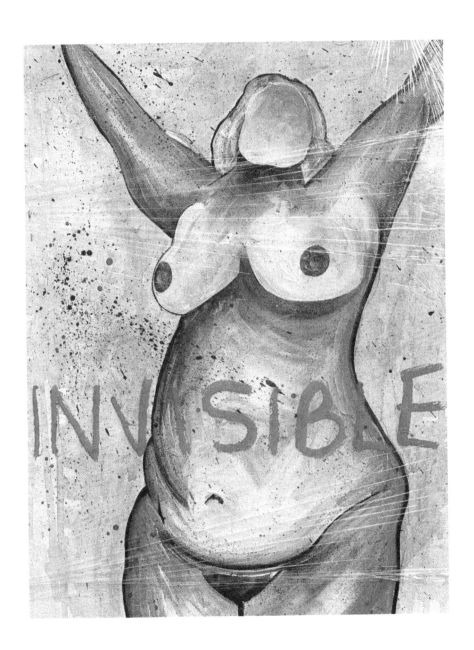

# *Stay Alive*

## Kay Louise Aldred


6.30 am alarm.
Kids out of bed – breakfast – dressed – teeth brushed – school.
8 am work meeting.
"Stay Alive!" shouts the pain.
Teach 3 lessons.
12.30 pm lunch meeting.
"Fight back" – "Demand rest" it barks.
"Refuse to do anymore" it insists.
Teach 2 lessons.
4 pm work meeting.
"Say no" – "You're not listening" – "Ok, lets try a different way"
Nausea. Aching. Bloating. Swelling. Throbbing. Heat. Dizziness.
Pounding, searing, fire balls.
Razor cutting right-hand side sensation.
Blinded, zig zag lines.
I can't see the computer screen. Do the work later tonight.
5.30 pm Home.
Pain onslaught. Vomit.
6-9 pm.
Kids' homework – tea – bath – story – goodnight kiss.
9.30 pm.
Need to prepare for tomorrow.
11 pm
Lie down.
"Stay Alive" – it whispers.

# *Kali*

## Michelle Moirai

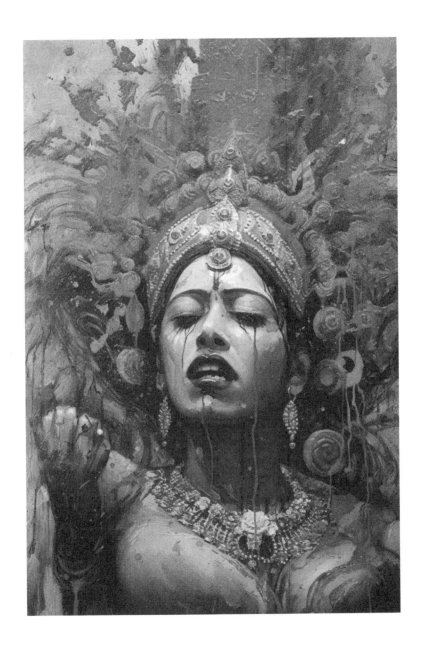

# The Patriarchal Healthcare System

Siobhan Finnegan

There has been a recent resurgence in feminist science writers and journalists exposing medical injustices against women. These include Maya Dusenbury's work on the many ways in which women's pain is dismissed and their testimonies discredited, to Caroline Criado-Perez's findings on the Data Gap in healthcare research for women's bodies and their healthcare needs. To the new work by Sarah Graham, in her book Rebel Bodies, where she calls for Gender Health Care Revolution. It is beginning to feel that we are moving toward a critical mass of dissenting voices around the many ways in which women are mistreated under Patriarchal Healthcare Institutions.

Ashley Fetters wrote in *The Atlantic*[9] about the dismissal of women's sexual or reproductive health concerns as 'healthcare-gaslighting'. The term 'medical-gaslighting' has also been used to illustrate this phenomenon. Though, it is not only women's sexual health that is a neglected area of research and care, the whole 'care' system is steeped in deeply misogynistic attitudes. From the devaluation care work, which is underpaid and usually the domain of working class or immigrant women. To the under acknowledged and under researched bodies of women in all healthcare disciplines. Through the positioning of the desirable 'norm' as male, white, fit, young, heterosexual body. Which becomes the marker from which all other bodies are measured against and therefore become both deviant and deviated from.

The institutions of health care and medicine do not exist in a vacuum, they are steeped in patriarchal economic and political aims and objectives. They also come with the ghosts of colonial history. It would appear that we are yet to shake off Darwin's

---

[9] printed on 10/08/18.

assumptions which position women as biologically and intellectually inferior to men (Saini 2017. Pg 19). When you have a dominant, partial view that positions itself as the knower of the things to be known. That creates logic, sciences, laws, narratives, economic systems, and other ideas – that prop up and reinforce its position, whilst demonizing, subordinating, and ridiculing any bodies or forms of knowledge that may challenge its hold on power. Which in turn produces chronic imbalances of health, wealth, and broader ecological and environmental matters.

This lobsided view of everything, which has been centuries in the making, can be unpacked in several ways. With regards to chronic health conditions, which under this rubric, are individualized into 'something wrong with the person' rather than explored systemically as 'something wrong with the environment, in which this person is moving through'. The environment being a heterosexist, patriarchal, white supremist, ablest society, that is currently enacting an ecocide, that I suggest, can be felt, not only in the changes in the climate, the land, the seas, and animals, but in our bodies.

Female Bodies are immediately othered as soon as they put one foot through the door of a medical doctor's office, they become an object of curiosity, a statistic, or an interesting case at best, dismissed as a hysteric or time waster at worst (Dusenbery 2018). Medical training requires one to have authoritative knowledge of the patient's body. This way of thinking can be traced back to the European colonial projects which also saw the implementation of royal institutions of medical bodies. The embodiment of the 'rational' 'civilized' professionalized subject can be seen in Said's (2003) observations of how the British Colonials viewed themselves in relation to Arabic nations. They created the term Oriental, to which they declared that they knew 'Orientals' better than they knew themselves. It brings to mind the doctor patient relationship, to which the doctor assumes the knowledge over the patient, 'doctor knows best'.

This colonial, medical, scientific gaze also determined the taxonomy of plant specimens, the classification and measurement bodies that could be divided into races, which produced assumptions about temperament and evolutionary status, without the need for dialogue and engagement with native subjects (McClintock's 1995). These colonial bodies, the bodies of the Enlightenment thinkers and the institutional bodies of medical societies produced particular hierarchies and power structures through the privileging of 'knowledge' espoused by them. Designating who has the authority to name what or whom. Creating an environment of who can speak on behalf of whom, of where 'objectivity' lies, who is the subject and becomes subjugated by it through the medical gaze (Foucault 2003).

This detachment or dualism is further enhanced by the influence of mechanism and its 'ontology of death', Foucault and Engelhardt observed a shift in the eighteenth century away from a symptom experience assessment, towards the knowledge of the corpse (Leder 1992). The physician's 'superior' observation skills and the pathologist's knife became the main implements of assessment (Leder 1992). Harding (1991) and Haraway (1988) also observed this privileging of the eye under the medical gaze, the view from nowhere, that of white upper/middle class male, that is ungendered, unraced, unreflective of itself, not situated anywhere and therefore unaccountable. Haraway (1988) notes how the privileging of the eye extends to that of satellites, cameras, MRIs, X-rays and so on, making vision superior. But a vision that has been designed through dualistic medial gaze which is limited and reductive. The colonizer's gaze, as Spiller (2013) points out, was a practice that dismissed and ridiculed the African's knowledge as inferior. Knowledge that was gained through touch, feeling and healing. A knowledge made inferior, which was to be associated with the emotional or feminine, not quantifiable or able to stand up against rigorous measures of medical testing. An affective knowledge which is very much diminished through the process of medical training; studies demonstrate declining levels of empathy, to be replaced by 'detached concern' (Elton 2018), or made obscure by the performed 'bedside manner'. None of which aids communication, opens dialogue or a felt sense, but rather produces a bizarre macabre performance between the assessor and those to be assessed, that is the medical encounter.

As with Barad's (2007) apparatus of the 2-slit experiment in quantum physics, something changes for/within the patient under the medical gaze. In this case, there is a lost connection, a disavowal of the person under the guise of the 'rational' doctor. A process not dissimilar to Fanon's (2017) 'crushing objecthood', the patient is reminded of their inferiority every time they enter the space of the medical encounter. I would also suggest that it produces dissociative effects within doctors and healthcare professionals. This could be countered by an insightful doctor or health professional, but my experience of this is far and few between. Because the doctor or health professional tends to (dis)embody the dysfunctions of a Patriarchal healthcare system as they become (un)witting perpetrators of the structural violence embedded within it.

Caroline Elton (who provide counselling for doctors) and Nathalie Martinek (who critiques the cultures in medical institutions) talk about how medical school is traumatising – it functions like military indoctrination to de-empathize, detach and fragment the medical students. It is not only patients who suffer in these environments, with around 45% of junior doctors quitting their chosen profession each year. Martinek discusses in her work, that what hides behind the conveniently individualising term, 'Burn Out' is actually assimilation trauma, or moral injury trauma. Those who have a greater moral compass will suffer in these places, and those who are focused on power, whether it is the acquisition of it or the adherence to it, will both maintain the status quo and knowingly or unknowingly continue to perpetuate structural violence of this patriarchally influenced culture.

Medical training has a tendency to position the doctor as valid, rational, knower and the patient as the invalid, irrational, object to be known. Which is why they can't handle it if the object speaks, so they dismiss the object, the object justifiably becomes distressed and the knower is then satisfied with their initial judgement, as they can now place the object into the preprepared trop of emotional and irrational. Thus, absolving themselves from all forms of reflective practice and accountability.

And of course, if the doctor gets emotional (read angry, dismissive, sarcastic and defensive), it is also the patient's fault for 'non-compliance', 'treatment seeking', 'obstinance' and whatever old othering claptrap they can use to gaslight, derail and generally confuse and invalidate the patient. As these interactions are so common for many women seeking healthcare, they become part of the wallpaper. Repeated so much, they seem normal; to be expected and accepted. We don't have an agreed understanding with contextual circumstances to identify and name these behaviours as unacceptable and potentially harmful. Such as in the way the term Sexual Harassment provided communication and legislation to identify forms of assault and intimidation, women previously had no words to collectively describe.

Concepts such as Miranda Fricker's work on Epistemological, Testimonial and Hermeneutical Injustices might provide the groundwork for this matter. Firstly, epistemological injustice refers to assumptions about knowledge, such as in *medical knowledge is always superior to patient knowledge*. As in 'doctor knows best', who are the knowers and who are the 'to be known', the 'objective', 'rational' gaze from nowhere. Secondly the testimony of the patient is often considered merely 'subjective', whilst often viewed as 'emotional', 'irrelevant', 'manipulative' or 'problematic'. This perception is increased double-fold if the patient represents what is to be consider a less reliable or credible social group. Whilst hermeneutical injustice stems from the lack of access, capacity or opportunity to knowledge that could help you or others to understand your/their situation. Examples of this could include not having access to your medical notes, not understanding the language used to describe healthcare matters, or not having information about the contextual culture where certain relational power dynamics might be restricting one's access to the best care and treatment.

By creating terms to identify the violence created under these patriarchal institutions, we could also offer up some alternatives to more effective care systems.

Judith Herman (2015) recommends body orientating therapeutic interventions and is a firm believer that politics cannot be separated from therapeutic or medical processes. She came out of a background of civil rights movements and was also an activist in the women's movement. This viewpoint gave her the opportunity to observe a broader epidemic of both physical and structural violence against oppressed groups. Her experience in consciousness-raising spaces taught her to trust the personal testimonies of women, not to pathologize these people, but rather to contextualize their experiences. She also observed how the institutions set up to provide care for people re-enacted the abuse through denial of their experiences.

Blackman (2008) discusses a return to the body, the somatically felt body, for which she references Tamborinino's description of gut feelings, intelligence of the flesh and an attunement with our encounters and interactions. This is like Barad's (2003) material agency. These bodily, material agencies will make themselves known in whatever way they can. But if Patriarchal cultures have interrupted the process through the trauma-inducing, agential cutting systems, the message or communication may have to move forcefully to be heard. Blackman (2008) refers to the work of Bordo who draws on the Foucauldian concepts of the 'docile body, bio-power and micro practices of self and social regulation'. She discusses Bordo's work with women's relationship with food as a denial of the body, constituted by the Cartesian dualism, mind over matter. Patriarchy is the water we swim in and if we do not have the language to identify it, it will tell us that we and our bodies are the problem. We are too much and not enough it will say.

The journey of returning to the body, as Donna Haraway would say, is to stay with the trouble, bear witness to the senses, to the discomfort, to the pain. To learn the language of the body and all the memories it holds is not an easy task in this Patriarchal culture as we have been conditioned to moralise over bodily sensations rather than listen, connect, and enter dialogue with these old wisdoms.

This practice of attempting to devalue the knowledge of somatic sensations and emotional intelligence (not the sort that requires the controlling or manipulation of emotions, but rather the one that feels into and listens to emotions) creates a barrier to communication. Being able to listen requires empathy; if doctors cannot effectively listen or practice humility we are in an extremely dangerous situation. This goes for healthcare professionals of all genders working in a culture that focuses more on 'rational expertise' over 'embodied care and knowing'.

References

Barad, K. (2007) Meeting the Universe Halfway: Duke University Press.

Barad, K (2003) Posthumanist Performativity: Towards an Understanding of How Matter Come to Matter (Signs: Journal of Woman in Culture and Society 2003, vol 28, no. 3).

Blackman, L. (2012) Immaterial Bodies. Affect, Embodiment and Mediation. Nottingham. Sage.

Blackman, L. (2008) The Body. The key concepts. Oxford. Berg Bordo, S. (2004). Unbearable weight. Berkeley, Calif: Univ of California Press.

Dusenbery, M. (2018) *Doing Harm; The truth about how bad medicine and lazy science leave women dismissed, misdiagnosed, and sick.* USA: Harper Collins.

Criado Perez, C. (2019) *Invisible Women. Exposing data bias in a world designed for men.* London. Vintage.

Elton, C. (2018). Also Human. London: William Heinemann. Fanon, F. (2017). Black Skin, White Masks. UK: Pluto Press.

Fetters, Ashley (2018) How Women's 'Health-Care Gaslighting' went mainstream - *The Atlantic*. http://www.theatlantic.com/family/archive/2018/08/womens-health-care-gaslighting/567149/

Foucault, M. (2003). *The Birth of the Clinic.* UK. Routledge Classics.

Fricker, Miranda (2007) *Epistemic Injustice. Power and the Ethics of Knowing.* NY, USA. Oxford University Press.

Graham, Sarah. (2023) Rebel Bodies, *A guide to the gender health gap revolution.* London. Greentree, Bloomsbury Publishing Plc

Harding, S. G. (1991). *Whose science? Whose knowledge?* Ithaca, N.Y: Cornell University Press.

# *Missing the Garden*

## Barbara O'Meara

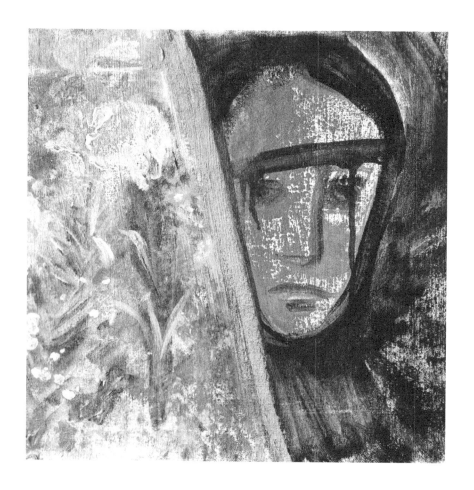

# Mother, Fire, Son

## Kohenet Dr. Harriette Wimms

All that I am is pain.
I come to, looking down at my body,
consciousness is my enemy
in this post-Cesarean moment,

rising to the surface of a narcotic river,
gasping and sputtering:
*Help!*

Wires, bags, monitors:
beeping, dripping, flashing.

The sound of emptiness,
respirations tighten, then loosen around my limbs.

The sterile room reeks of alcohol
and the nurse's compassion fatigue.

I am trapped. My captor's language is no
longer my own.

Listen to me please. I can feel it.
I can feel the cut. Please help me, please.

> *You are so dramatic.*
> *You tell me it hurts,*
> *I give you more morphine,*
> *then you pass out.*
> *You don't hurt. You are fine.*

What? I don't understand... and where is my baby, anyway?
This isn't how it happens in the movies:

this is not all pants and pushes.
*It's a boy, cut the cord*—skin-to-skin bliss.
This is fire and brimstone.

My arms: empty and strapped down.
IVs in the tender blue tracks on the back of both hands,
my blood pushing up against the fluid.
Shivering and on my own. *I hate this.*

When they pulled him from me,
my body disappeared; I passed out.
The resident, kneeling on the stretcher,
following the doctor's order to use her full weight
against my ribs, disappearing my womb,
trying to force the baby out.
But he kept swimming away
in the expansive ocean of my uterus.

Is this how it ends?
Death after giving birth?
Am I even still breathing? Am I already gone?
The pain is a blinding light. White! Silver!
Gravity has forsaken me.
The cot beneath me hot with cold.
My hands tremble, search for my infant.
He belongs to the earth now.

I remember my friend peeking her head into recovery.
Smiling, simpering, taking a breath in
to utter something sickeningly sweet about a perfect baby.
I cut her off: Help me please. I can't stand the pain.

The day my son was born, 6 hours passed before I held him in my
arms.

Puzzled by my escalating diastolic and systolic, the nurse explained,

> *We can't let you leave here until you calm yourself*
> *and bring that pressure down.*

Idiot!

I remember pain pulsing in my ears
from my brand spanking new, bright red
Cesarean-section;
the day my son was born.

When finally, I wrapped my arms around
the howling mouth, the moon face, the tightened body—
my pain became a sacrifice at Shekhinah's altar.
A sacred smoke: my message to The Divine.
And the pain disappeared when I held him, at last, in my arms.
He stopped crying, too.

I remember the first moment I held my son, my baby lion,
I touched the generations past and yet to come.
The day he was born, I became a phoenix.
We continue to soar.

# *Becoming Morrigan*

Barbara O'Meara

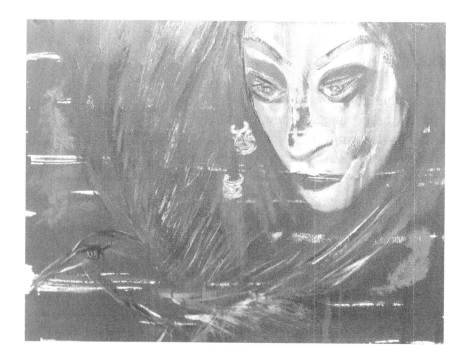

# The Truth in Pain

## Sionainn McLean

No man would ever be told to take an ibuprofen before getting a biopsy on their uterine lining. The closest equivalent I can think of that a man might have to endure in comparison is a colonoscopy. And that's not the best example, and women endure that procedure as well. There's just no comparison really.

If you are triggered by pap smears, stop reading now. But we know that feeling. Laying on the table, legs spread with a paper cloth draped unceremoniously over our lower half. Scootch, we're told. Does anyone get the position right on the first try? Sometimes my legs are "manually" moved, spread a bit wider. There's an unceremonious insertion – it's cold, and most times, enough lube to create a slip and slide, though when there's not, you know it. It always hurts though, for me.

Relax.

Particularly from women gynecologists, I have to ask… do you really think telling me to relax helps? Memories of assault come up. Fears of it happening again. I recall when I gave birth to my first child, an aged old man who still asked his nurses to shave women giving birth "for hygiene" who stripped me of my own bodily autonomy, reducing me to a vessel carrying the most sacred of life – my own life barely a thought.

Pain is just part of being a woman. It just seemed to go hand in hand, I've never had anyone say this to me, it was just always there. Our first time "hurts" is the standard mythology. Childbirth is the most beautiful pain, and women who choose not to feel that pain are looked down upon. Women who choose to feel it are crazy. We're damned if we do, damned if we don't.

Chronic pain is a smile while holding back tears. "I'm fine. Just tired. What do you need? How can I help?" I tell the world.

Chronic pain is shouting "I'm a bad ass woman!" with all the other warrior women, but inside, feeling as though you are weak, and are about to come undone. Chronic pain is crying behind closed doors as you lose another friend, another opportunity, your momentum, and a sense of a promising future.

This was me.

Until one day, in a haze of tears, depression, anxiety and pain that felt like a knife in my joints – my aching hip, my fingers barely able to move, my back radiating agony, all on top of the cramping from my period, my breasts feeling like they were someone's punching bag, and my jaw/neck/head linked pain making me wish for death. Brigid sat in front of me.

"It's time to do something." She told me. She had flaming red hair, gentle green eyes, though she also looked like a friend I knew. She put her hands around me, and the pain eased. "This isn't something you have to live with." She reminded me.

But what could I do. I didn't ask, I sat there, sort of resigned. Brigid was wrong. I was a woman. No one cared about my pain because I was a woman. This pain was in my head. It was... my punishment for failures, for not being a super mom, super wife, super woman. For being weak.

A crow flew in and landed on Brigid's shoulder. "I told you, she's stubborn. Let me help." I knew that voice, that crow. She flew at me and began to peck. The pain rose again. I wanted to stop her, but she yelled, firmly. "Don't fight me."

The Morrigan pecked at me, tearing my wounded, and rotting flesh. I sobbed and screamed, and then I went silent. Thoughts floated by, one by one until there was nothing but darkness. I looked at my body, from outside of it. It was ripped into shreds, bone exposed. The Morrigan was without mercy, I thought. But then I noticed the flesh that did remain. It was the healthy flesh. She left me there, my decaying bits consumed. "Brigid will tend to you for now."

Brigid lay beside my body. It reminded me of those scenes in movies where two friends sit beneath the open sky. Only the sky was like an aurora, with whole galaxies swirling, shooting stars. The air smelled like cinnamon, and lavender, and rosemary. Brigid only sat up once, laying her mantle over me.

"It's time to heal," She said. Her voice was softer now, gentler. "This pain is not something to endure. It's telling you truths. Truths you want to ignore."

"This pain is not punishment."

"This pain is not because you are a woman. It's not in your head, it's very, very real."

"This pain is sacred, but not in the way you think." I find myself lifting an arm, to try to touch a shooting star. I'm listening to her, but I can't help but notice the way it looks. I'm feeling my body as my mind feels the Universe around me. Her warmth, her compassion, her healing is radiating through both, and while the tears are not stopping, it's all a release. My arm, a mix of bone and sinew and flesh, is healing before me. I am raw, but whole.

"This pain is telling you to change. That something is wrong." Brigid continues. I hear footsteps, and yet another Goddess is there. Herbs are sprouting from my body, and she's gathering them. Airmid doesn't speak to me, but her smile is gentle.

"This pain is telling you that you hold too much within yourself." Brigid continues. "You have to let go of it." I think back, remember all the times I've done just that. Held it in, negative feelings, pain, disappointment, frustration. Fear.

"This pain won't just go away, but it can get better." Brigid is laying her hands over me, and it hurts again, but in a different way. This is the pain of growth, of realization, of my own power coming into place. "You have more control than you think." Airmid leaves a chamomile flower on my chest.

"Start there."

There were many realizations for me. There was a lot of healing after. Am I perfect? Has the pain gone away? No, but I do what I can. I show myself compassion and gentleness. I take baby steps still. One thing at a time, one day at a time, and some days, I really feel overwhelmed. The Morrigan reminds me not to expect perfection – that expectation leads to rotting, and she will tear that out of me if I let it settle within myself. Brigid reminds me that if I don't tend to my body and my mind – which are the things I can most control, then I can't continue to heal. I will be growing and healing until my last breath. Airmid reminds me that I'm not alone. Not only do I have the goddesses beside me, but I have herbal friends and spiritual allies. The chamomile was her reminder that I had to de-stress. Since then, she's introduced me to many herbal friends to aid me.

I go about my days now trying my best. If my body hurts, which it does often, I listen and I rest, and take care of myself. I try to eat healthier. I try to move more. Blood flow, it seems is good for my body, particularly in places like my hips. I de-stress A LOT. I drink herbal teas, I meditate, I reflect in my journals. My place in this world is temporary, but that doesn't mean I should not tend to my temple, my body. I revere it, even when I'm angry with it. I don't succumb to the foolish notion that somehow as a woman, this pain isn't real, that it's all in my head, or that it's some sort of punishment for imperfection. I fight to be heard. I've fired my medical team and found one that doesn't dismiss me.

Does the pain suck? Yes. Don't let anyone tell you otherwise. You don't deserve pain. The Goddess doesn't want you to be in pain. Sometimes, that's just a part of the human condition. And that's hard to face, I know. You deserve treatment, and while sometimes there may not be a treatment, you still have things you can control to help ease the pain. Mostly, you can show yourself compassion. Rest. Relax – make it a priority, and do so without guilt, no matter what others might say. Don't be afraid of the word no. And don't hold it in. Even when you think the world is looking down on you, telling you that you must endure, that it's just part of "being a woman", and the world can't stop just because you are in pain – they are wrong. Rest and self-care is not stopping, it's treatment, it's healing and you are so worthy of that.

# *Brigid*

## Barbara O'Meara

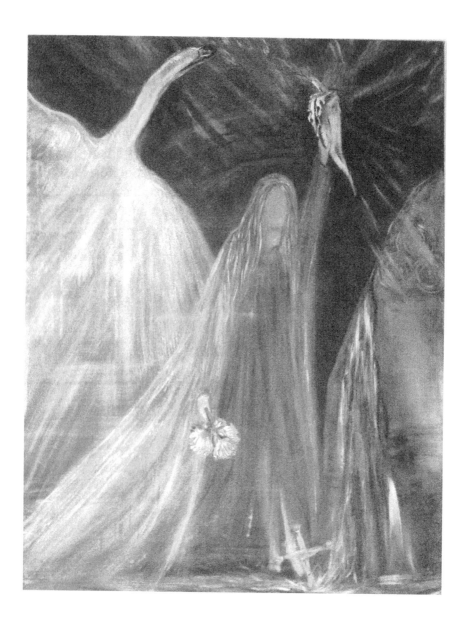

# The Pain of Missing
# The Hope of Goddess

### Jeanine E. Otte

How do I measure the pain of a missing Self?
The fever from an untended Flame?
The cavity inside mothers I absorbed as a girl?

Do I count the sighs I ate for breakfast that mother served me
with my cereal?
Or is it in the depths of her sighs?
Did the breath reach her toes as her body ached for paths
un-walked?
Did the air tickle her lungs reaching for the voice unspoken?
Unspoken by her?
Unspoken by her mother?

Do I measure the ever-present timber of my father-pastor's
voice?
The tacit domination,
The prayers absent of Feminine Power, absent of Me?

How do I describe an agony so present yet evasive in name?
How do I nourish an organ that no one told me existed?
How do I name the pain so I can heal?

Is it in the grinding teeth that eroded my enamel?
The TMJ that sears my jaw, my temples, in middle age?

Is it in the bitterness of domestication?
The harrowing depression of give, give, give?
The unclaimed desire of the wet between my legs?

How do I name something so inside of myself that I never once heard uttered by the
mothers,
grandmothers,
aunts?
Let alone the
fathers,
grandfathers,
uncles?

Perfectionism, whiteness, religiosity. Self-denial disguised as truth.

As a child I caught glimpses of Goddess royalty
in wild mushroom caps carefully collected and framed on living rooms walls.
in chatter over freshly brewed coffee during playtime.
in soft hands on my back at bedtime.
in questions about male gods in Sunday school.
in red teenage girl rage at men's abuse.
in the Old Tree Bridge that carried our imaginations, our sparks.

To heal, I lay down with my child to listen, to find a balm for an unnamed wound.

Relief manifests in dreams with my grandmother – emerging when the tightrope from the male ego dance begins to stiffen around my neck.

She appears to say
    Cut the rope.
    It is You.
    It is All of Us.
    Be Free.

She is the Crow who rescues me from a false sanctuary and turns my robe from white to black.
She is the Rainbow hue of a doe looking upon me in the thick of the woods.
She is the young Girl floating peacefully in a cool pond among prairie grass.

She is the Serpent circling me in water awaiting my transformation.

She is Mother donning a royal gold gown and bearing a staff, inviting me to walk within the crook of Her arm.

She is Lilith leaving stone houses of ingratitude and disrespect.

She is Inanna changing
        ingratitude to celebration
        disrespect to reverence
        death to reBirth.

To Goddess from whom all Life emerges and evolves and story and Mystery.

To I, to She, to We.

To Us.
To Always and Infinite Spirals of Light and Dark.
May we see the Dreams of our Grandmothers.
May we hear the Wisdom of our Children.
May we delight in the sustenance of Earth and give Her sustenance in return.
May we rise as the Queens We Are.
May We Heal.
May it be so for you.
May it be so for me.
May it be so for all of us.

# Finding Meaning in the Fire: Explaining Unexplained Chronic Pain

## Kay Louise Aldred

I've deciphered the mystery of the unexplained fire of chronic pain I experience. I've discovered the meaning of it. Access to the panacea for women's suffering and oppression. That's the explanation.

The cause of the fire:

1. Patriarchal structures
2. Patriarchal paradigms
3. Patriarchal conditioning
4. Patriarchal society

The meaning – the panacea:

1. Pleasure
2. Orgasms
3. Freedom
4. Choice
5. Creativity
6. Community
7. Support
8. Love
9. Shared responsibility of household tasks and childcare
10. Rest and support when grieving, after giving birth, during menstruation and during the menopause transition

It's quite simple really.

# Pain Perspectives

## Tamara Albanna

I've been living with chronic pain for as long as I can remember.

But it seems to be that at a particular point in my life, when I turned 13 and started menstruating, that the pain intensified. As a 44-year-old woman now who is in the throes of perimenopause, I have been able to make that connection, the root of the pain.

13 was not a good year. I grew up in an abusive household, and my mother used religious oppression to keep us (girls) in check, so when I began bleeding, what little freedoms I had were stripped from me. I was no longer swimming at the local pool all summer, my shorts and skirts got longer, and my overall behavior was scrutinized meticulously. Over time, I was made virtual prisoner in my own home, and learned to somehow exist in this situation, while watching my school friends mature and enjoy their increasing freedoms as they grew.

It truly was a curse, in every sense of the word, my monthly cycle. Instead of honoring that sacred time, it caused be pain, both physical and emotional. I blamed it for my imprisonment, and it seemed to fight back, every month.

I was bleeding, it was my responsibility to not tempt men. My body was sinful, my biology was sinful. As a woman I was simply damned. Except, I wasn't even a woman yet. My childhood and adolescence stripped from me.

Then the migraines started.

That was an entire new level of hell that I hadn't endured prior.

They were debilitating, bringing me to my knees each time, with pain so bad I wished for death some nights. When my father realized I might be ill, (it took a few years), I was taken to the family doctor for a scan. It was clear, I was given medication and it didn't work.

Our doctor, an Iraqi man of course who I expected would tell my parents everything, pulled me aside and asked what was going on. I lied and said, "nothing." What was he going to do for me anyway? I was 16, and things were only getting worse.

The compounding of physical and emotional pain, an abusive household, and religious trauma was far too much to bear. I checked out of my body. The pain would come and I would take as many pills as I could and try to sleep through it.

In hindsight, I probably lost years of life lying in bed, wishing for an end.

My body was screaming at this point, I wasn't listening.

I got married, the pain endured. I had children, the pain endured.

It was relentless, no end in sight. I remained in deep disconnect. I lost time with my children, spent days laying in a hotel bed instead of out enjoying a vacation, sleeping through holidays, and just losing precious time I can never get back, struggling through pain.

It wasn't until I reached my 40s that I was able to deconstruct what had happened to me fully. The way I was taken out of my body by patriarchy, by Abrahamic faith that disconnected me from the Goddess, blood, and life. I was life, I bled. It was not dirty, it should not be hidden, it was not wrong.

I remember hearing or reading somewhere that the Goddess requires no sacrifice because we bleed monthly. Instead of being blessed, I spent my life feeling cursed. I remember being told I was "unclean" and therefore banned from prayers during religious holidays when I bled. Fuck you and your male god. The Goddess would have us bleed into the earth as an offering.

The older I get, and the closer to the Crone I am, I mourn the Maiden who never was, and the Mother who struggled. But I tell my story to save other women and girls this very real pain I endured, that many endure.

My migraines are less frequent now. After different treatments, a good old piercing seemed to do the trick (in both ears) as well as an IUD. Every woman is different, we cope differently, we find ways to manage, to minimize suffering.

Mothers, teach your daughters well, remind them who they are. Remind them who they come from, that their blood is sacred. That pain serves as a reminder oftentimes that we have in fact lost ourselves.

# *Internal Combustion*

Traci Purwin

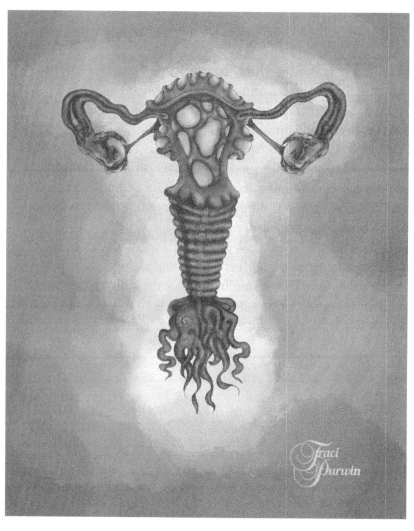

Medium: Digital Painting
Inspiration: My love hate relationship with my womb. I have polycystic ovarian syndrome, and some days I feel as though it's a spaceship invading my body.

# Dancing Wind

Laura Valenti

**Hard times require furious dancing. ~Alice Walker**

*Below is part of my story where I share my journey with cancer, depression and suicidal tendencies. Please ensure you are in a good place when you read it and know I am not offering medical advice here.*

I don't like labels.

But recently, I have been wondering whether it would help me put things in perspective and be more accepting if I said that I've lived with chronic depressive states throughout my life. Interestingly enough, I am editing this piece while embracing my journey with osteoarthritis.

My health, in one way or another, has always been my Achilles' heel.

I was isolated in a hospital for a week or two when I was only two months old. I had a contagious skin infection that was about to dangerously attack my internal organs.

By age five, I suffered from malabsorption and developed ongoing immunity issues.

I remember being in love with the dance since I was a child.

I also remember knowing everything was alive: the trees, the flowers, the mountains, and the sea.

I lived with my dad and grandparents in a small conservative town near Rome.

My mum died suddenly from a brain aneurysm when I was six. She was only thirty-four years old.

I have a blurred memory of that day. She had to pick me up from my grandparents' home but never showed up so my dad came to pick me up instead. When we returned to our flat, he opened the door and noticed something was off in the apartment. He quietly asked me to visit the neighbours. I can't recall exactly what happened because I have memory gaps from that time. But I remember a terrifying sense of confusion and despair. Children are very intuitive. I knew in my being that something terrible had happened.

I spent a few days with the neighbours and didn't attend my mum's funeral. My dad told me that she was in the hospital and she might be back. He forbade my other relatives to tell me that she was dead. I think he was so broken he did not know how to cope with a little girl who lost her mum. The only person I would go to was my beloved grandfather. I would tell him I wanted my mum. When I think about it, I can feel his heart breaking. Looking back, I can sense how his love kept me (relatively) sane and alive.

My dad told me that Mum was dead after over a month.

As a young adult, I often feared that I was going mad. I also felt suicidal many times. In a way, I knew I would not take my life. But I often struggled with why I was experiencing those states full of despair.

I grew up in a household where there was a lot of yelling. My father often beat me, belittled me and said cynical words that left me ashamed, paralysed and terrified. My little heart was crushed many times. I now know that my nervous system was constantly on hyperarousal, scanning for danger. I felt unsafe, unseen and unloved and developed the belief that something was wrong with me early on. All the above was also very confusing because I loved my dad dearly; he was all I had. To forgive (and not condone) him has been one of the greatest lessons in my life.

Today, I feel much love, tenderness and compassion for that little girl who still lives inside me.

As a child, I used to lock myself in the living room, put the stereo at high volume, and shake my body until I was exhausted (listening to heavy metal music!) I still remember my grandmother storming into the room and shouting to put the volume down, worried about what the neighbours would think. I instinctively found a way to cope, live and find relief: I used to go bananas and dance my socks off! There was a primal, earthy intelligence moving through my body. I was intuitively releasing stress or simply sensing a part of me that was alive, healthy, wild, passionate and curious. Those were my first encounters with the Divine.

Dance became my medicine.

The Cosmic Mother wanted me to move, shake, leap, and sweat. I would spontaneously enter altered states of consciousness and trance where I could experience a sense of communion with all life. There was no trauma, worry or drama there. Only the joy of my dancing animal body.

By age ten, I was already smoking, bleeding, and kissing. Many mothers did not want their kids to hang out with me as I was a bad influence. As a teenager, I started taking many drugs and developed a self-destructive drive. I disliked myself and my body. I medicated myself with substances and food. My first boyfriend beat me up and left me with black eyes and bruises all over my body. I was scarred emotionally and at the soul level. My self-esteem went under my feet. I guess I had a distorted idea about love and had no clue how to take care of myself kindly. I probably felt that I deserved to be treated in that way.

On the other hand, another part of me was very hungry for life, adventure, magic and meaning. I became fascinated with physical movement because it allowed me to express myself, feel creative and lighter and liberate some burdens too unfathomable to be spoken about.

I loved to dance. I admired those who fought for freedom and those who overcame adversities and transformed their pain into medicine and wisdom. And I loved the poets, the writers, the artists, the wounded healers, the medicine women, the priestesses, the magicians, the alchemists, the Earth protectors, the dancers, the activists and the rebels. I wanted to be one of them. And I did not want to turn bitter.

**In my chaotic years at university, I discovered my love for the drums.**

Whenever there was a drummer, I would appear next to him or her, leaping, abandoning myself to the dance. My body would relax into the beat and rhythm, connecting to the ground and the Earth. As a young adult, I intuitively knew that I had experienced states of dissociation many times. Some call it soul loss. Part of me was living up in the clouds.

Without formal training or education in holistic health or somatics or movement, I knew I longed to return home to my body, as it was my sacred temple. When I danced, my body could spontaneously relax, bend, spiral, and twist, and I could tap into ancient inner wisdom. It was a form of soul retrieval. I could express, move and liberate stuck energies. I was an expression of the pulse of the Cosmic Mother and Divine intelligence.

I did not consciously know I was looking for the Divine Mother when I was younger. But I was, always.

I was looking for Her in every drop of alcohol I ingested. I was looking for the Divine, the sacred and a glimpse of ecstasy. I searched in every stranger's eyes, my dog's warm affection, teachers whom I put on a pedestal, and a lover's harsh words.

I was starved for love. I developed various forms of addiction to fill the void I felt inside. I was looking for roots.

There was so much self-hatred and self-rejection inside me. Paradoxically, I also had a strong compulsion to feel important because, probably secretly, I believed I did not matter.

I searched for external validation and answers. I often put my life in danger. And I allowed people to treat me like a doormat.

Occasionally, I would find the Divine Mother as an expression of self-acceptance and compassion in the beat, my hips and feet, the music, the rhythm and wild dances, and the long nights I spent outdoors staring at the Moon and the Stars. Sometimes, walking in a forest or on a beach, I would feel that even if I was wounded, I was a walking miracle and part of something bigger than me, mysterious, sacred and magical. I give thanks for the times I could sit in awe and bow to life.

A few weeks after attending a very intense Movement Medicine workshop in my early thirties, a lump suddenly started growing at the heart level on my chest. I literally vomited it out. I am glad my body pushed it out so it became visible and did not kill me silently from the inside. A few weeks later, it was the size of an apple, and I could barely move. It was impossible to ignore it. This time, I had to listen. I was in pain, and doctors misdiagnosed me a few times, but my intuition kept telling me something was wrong. After going to several hospitals, I was diagnosed with non-Hodgkin's lymphoma. I was thirty-three years old. Mum died when she was thirty-four. Was all this a random occurrence?

I refused to see cancer as a curse. When I was diagnosed, I knew I had to learn to embrace myself with kindness, love, softness and self-acceptance. I surrendered to the fact that I needed support and was vulnerable. I prayed and asked for help from White Tara and Kwan Yin.

I decided this situation would be an adventure.

I immediately went to therapy, changed my diet, and interrupted communication with my family (as I needed to hold firm boundaries and put myself first). I prayed to Goddess Kali to give me the courage to do what was right for me, remove obstacles on my healing path and be assertive.

While I underwent chemo, I danced off my socks! I became a lover of ritual and attended countless healing ceremonies where I danced for hours, sometimes even days, with no substances involved.

The dance helped me stay strong and gave me many insights into my process and life. Most importantly, I could explore repressed emotions that needed expression through movement.

I imagined the Goddess would want me to feel sensual and enjoy myself even if I struggled. She wanted me to move and 'sequence' out of my body undigested stuff.

The dance became a tool to bring to completion, symbolically, things that I could not do when I was younger.

Whenever I danced and discovered a new movement, I felt a sense of possibility and a fresh breeze. Through my whole body in motion, I could create new narratives that had nothing to do with being a victim or being powerless. I could become the thunder, the soft rain, the green moss, the rose, the tree, the eagle or the jaguar. I could sense my wings, roots, and the Goddess moving through me. I could hear the land whispering to me and, day by day, my soul landing more fully into my body. And more radically, I could feel pleasure, be playful and have fun! I named myself Dancing Wind.

I knew that for women under thirty-five, it was hazardous to combine chemotherapy and radiotherapy. When the hospital called me to follow the protocol and have radiotherapy, I refused and walked away. I could feel the strength I gathered thanks to the whole experience, people's support and many dances! The cancer was no longer active.

Shortly after the treatment, I separated from my boyfriend in London.

The pain was excruciating and overwhelming (as it triggered the wound of abandonment). I could barely function, sleep, eat and leave the floor for a few days.

I was tired and emotionally depleted and needed to rest and focus on the basics: eating, restoring and sleeping. I also longed deeply to sense the ground underneath me, the Earth and surrender. And so there I was, lying on the floor for days. I had very little stamina; all I could do was cry and ask for help from the Divine Mother. Once again, I was surrendering my pain to Her. I was paradoxically experiencing excruciating pain and having a sensual experience simultaneously.

I remember singing over and over the song: 'We all come from the Goddess, and to Her, we shall return like a drop of rain, falling into the Ocean. Hoof and horn, hoof and horn, all that dies shall be reborn. Wine and grain, wine and grain, all that falls shall rise again.' I must have sung it a hundred times.

I felt that my healing was the healing of the women in my lineage who came before me and were muted and lost their voices.

I was re-living the wound of abandonment. I was pissed at the Goddess. I felt lonely and lost. And I used to say: 'If you are really there, and I am meant to help others in their healing journeys because of this, please send me a sign because I am about to give up.'

Then little miracles would occur: a friend would call, or a fox would appear before my window.

I was not alone.

Resources:
The ACE study explores the effects of childhood adversities and how those impact long-term well-being and contribute to chronic illness. It considers these challenges a matter of public health.

# Deep Surrender

Arna Baartz

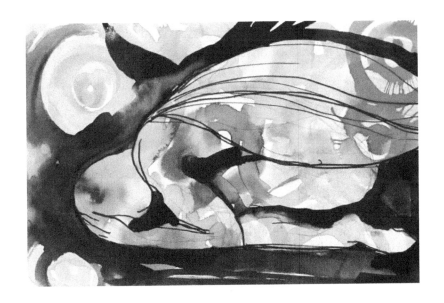

# *Dear Floor*

## Geo Bitgood

When I tell you that the floor is my best friend
You must know it was not always so

I pushed away; feared it; cursed it
"Please! anything but that!"

but always the return—
until it was... all there was

When you, your body, must meld and yield
When bone, through flesh, makes bruise,
and left nor right bring easeful breath
When nose to floorboard and eyes to ceiling
are bought by yowling blurry winces between

When floor is home
and bed,
and kitchen table,
and office,
and washroom,
and living room, all

When time defies sense, and place dwindles to one,
She is there for me.

As was involuntary, is now welcomed holding.
Gentle plane and gravity return me my newborn crawl

An inch of separation. Then two.
Then knee and hand, knee and hand and back again. To try again.

"Keep going."

So I do.
Until again I am able to take leave; never truly parted

I will see her again,
and in meanwhiles.

Each time, a lesser fear
Each time, a deeper memory of healing found anew

When I tell you that the floor is my best friend,
You must know it is with love and gratitude

# I Don't Slay the Dragon, I Am the Dragon

Iriome R. Martín Alonso

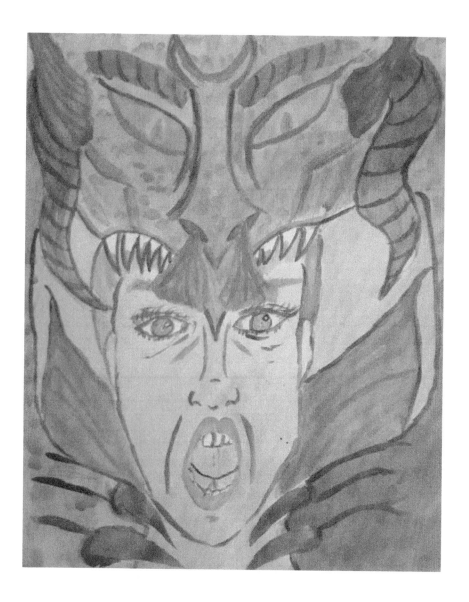

# Spear of Fire:
## The Healing and Burden of Fiery Names in Neurodivergent Minds

Iriome R. Martín Alonso

The concept of healing is bullshit.

Well, to some of us.

But let's rewind a bit, shall we?

My mother wanted to call me "Yavanna"[10]. To some of us this name is familiar; in Tolkien's *Silmarillion*, She's the Ainur/Valar – or what we could roughly translate as a "Goddess" of nature, specifically. My mother said that when she was pregnant she had a dream about me and she knew right there that *Yavanna* wasn't my name. She accepted my biological father's proposal instead – the only thing he gave me, besides life.

Hang in with me, I promise I'm getting somewhere here... but we need a tiny bit of context.

Iriome is an aboriginal name originating from the Canary Islands, which were conquered by the Europeans for almost a century between 1402 and 1496[11]. Currently, the world thinks of the Canary Islands as a tourist resort – knowing nothing about our past, culture, people or the consequences of colonialism that we still suffer from today. Some foreigners even dare to reclaim things they know nothing about. The Canary Islands are a bunch of Oceanic-African islands that still belong to Europe. We all descend from the Guanches who were raped, enslaved, tortured,

---

[10] Tolkien, J. R. R. (1977). *The Silmarillion*. George Allen & Unwin.
[11] Conquest of the Canary Islands. (2022, March 21). Wikipedia. https://en.wikipedia.org/wiki/Conquest_of_the_Canary_Islands

and murdered, and from the ones who did that to them, too. Back then, they stripped us from our tongue and we speak Spanish now. Some of us, however, carry aboriginal names.

Oral folklore tells us about a member of the noble class of the Guanches on the island of "La Palma" – which might sound familiar because it erupted horribly last year for months, taking people's homes and means of living – while mainlander Spanish folks and tourists came to collect lava ashes to sell on eBay, because contemporary colonialism doesn't exist at all...

As the legend goes, when Iriome's mother was pregnant, she couldn't think of any name was fit for the baby she was carrying. She was confident she would have a girl, so she prayed to the Goddess and asked Her to send her the name of her child in a dream. When she received the name, she knew her daughter would give meaning to it with her actions. Sadly, she didn't know how that would come to happen.

Months passed and her belly grew huge and heavy. She thought she would have a giant, or some sort of abnormal child, perhaps blessed or cursed by the Gods. When she was due, before the eyes of many, she unexpectedly gave birth to twins, a girl and a boy. But the Goddess had only sent her one single name, so she named them both the same[12].

It is said that we still know their names because they lived during the time of The Conquest and, as part of the warrior nobility, they both fought passionately against the invaders – together seemingly undefeatable, adding fire to their weapons to maximise their efforts against the conqueror's advanced war tactics and

---

[12] Currently "Iriome" is still a genderless or unisex name. The INE (Instituto Nacional de Estadística = National Institute of Statistics) tells us that there are 25 "women" with an average of 23,9 years and 306 "men" with the average of 12,6 years registered with the name "Iriome", which is funny if we think about the legend. As it is a Canary Island's aboriginal name (and pretty rare, may I add), it's safe to assume that this data is not only "national" but "international".
https://www.ine.es/widgets/nombApell/index.shtml

armament. Sadly, despite their courage and efforts to protect their land and people, the male twin was ultimately captured, enslaved and brought to Seville to be sold. She, on the other hand, powerless, saw everything that happened to her beloved brother and jumped from a cliff (we call that "enriscarse" from "risco," meaning "crag, cliff"), choosing death over becoming the slave of their enemies. The name, because of them, came to mean "Spear of Fire."

Gorgeous, right? Tragically beautiful, don't you think?

Well, I hated it.

Why in the world would someone choose a name for their child with such meaning and story? Well, my parents didn't know; that's my particular answer. Actually, my whole (long, very long) name meaning would roughly translate as "Spear of Fire of the Kings, God of War, Noble Warrior prepared to Fight."

Are you fucking serious? I'd much rather be called flower, lollipop, cloud. Urgh.

As a teenager, I hated my name. Most of my classmates had mainland Spanish names, or Guanche ones that were more common. I tried to shorten it to "Iry," spelled with an "y" because I thought it was "cooler." I tried different names – such as "Menty" or "Misty" (cringe), clearly influenced by Miley Cyrus' name change when she was a child. Essentially, I wanted anything that wasn't my name, but no name was as proper as Iriome was, either.

Names are shapeless, yet they somehow shape us. I'm not saying they determine us, Goddess forbid, but they end up meaning all that we are, they include the whole that's us. They're the invocation spell that summons us. For example, when I say "Coral" I think of the short, golden-blonde, greyish-green-eyed, kind woman that is my mother. Names are filled with meaning, with memories, with soul.

Just like in the stories, my mother didn't know how my full name would come to shape my life. I wish she had.

Do you know of something that is heavy, determining, undeniably there – but it's invisible too? Something that's forever, that never leaves, that will be there until your last breath on Earth? I do. It's called chronic mental illness.

We think of chronic fatigue, chronic asthma, chronic cardiomyopathy when we think of a chronic illness, but mental conditions can be forever, too, whether genetic or developed through trauma. And yes, you can get better, but some of us will never heal. And you know what? I don't blame myself for having asthma, I go swimming thrice a week to make it better, I do freediving, apnea breathing exercises, and train using singing and air control. I know I can never climb Mount Everest and I'm not interested in doing it. I know the limits of my chronic illness and I accept them. But it's harder, much harder, when mental disorders are involved.

Through all of my therapeutic processes, during all those years that I hated my name (just because I loathed myself and my name summarised who I was), I nurtured the all-devouring idea in my brain that I had to heal[13]. That I was going to the doctor to heal, that I was taking meds to heal, that I was going to the psychologist to heal. And to me a wound that healed was something ugly that *hurt*, a cut that closed and looked like nothing ever happened. Everything disappeared: the pain, the redness, the fear, the infection, the scar. Imagine a twelve-year-old girl's confusion when a wound she didn't see never disappeared, no matter what

---

[13]*Heal Verb.* (2022). Oxford Learners Dictionary. https://www.oxfordlearnersdictionaries.com/definition/english/heal?q=heal

she did or how much she tried, and it kept hurting, getting worse and worse.

Why couldn't I be whole again? Why couldn't I be pure, perfect, healed, untouched, immaculate? I didn't only carry the burden of my disorders, but also carried the guilt and shame of not recovering how I was "supposed to." It was like everyone expected me to stop being sick, to be who I was, or should have been, to just let it all go, but there was something that just didn't click. The guilt of being chronically ill with mental illness has probably hurt me more than the disorders my brain developed to survive.

My worst relapse was in September 2019. It fills me with sadness and rage how 22-year-old me tenderly thought, filled with hope, that she was healing, that she was "becoming normal." I could stop going to therapy weekly: My life was on track, I was properly diagnosed, the tools were more or less working; I let my guard down. The blow was horrible, it still persists.

I still don't fully accept that my life is somehow limited. I believe I'm the most worthless scum on Earth or an all-powerful monster wave, there's no in-between. A quarter century old woman, a twelve-year-old girl, who's told she's forever going to live with something that, at times, cripples her life – that limits her. Life is cruel. Nature is cruel. Goddess is cruel, and denying Her cruelty is like denying a hurricane's destruction. She's all, we're all Her, too.

Though my condition has been professionally diagnosed as severe, I have something called "concealed disorder" or "apparent functionality." It means that I organically mask my disorder in front of others, like a double protection mechanism. Essentially, people don't know that I'm going through it if I don't tell them, or unless they see me having a crisis. And I've felt so ashamed. My intelligence has been questioned; my abilities have been questioned. "She had so much potential" they say, as if I'm a perfect, broken doll, too damaged to be exposed and played with, suddenly useless.

People use it against you, too. No one is going to insult me by saying, "Hey, uh... she's got asthma, you know?" – but they have used my mental illness to discredit me in front of others when I haven't supported their questionable dynamics, cross of boundaries, ritual abuse, racism, xenophobia and trans exclusionary discourses. People who claimed to be there for me suddenly left without even asking my side of the story because the narrative was that I was "dangerous" and "crazy" – because I have a trauma-based illness they didn't know about, caused by someone who was not me, that they knew about from someone who wasn't me, while I actively worked on it with qualified specialists.

I wasn't the bright artist, the wise young priestess, or good loyal friend anymore; I was Iriome, the mentally ill girl who "could hurt you" even if her disorder forces her to hurt herself before daring to think about putting a hand on any other living creature. I've felt so betrayed. Would people have left me if I had cancer instead of a mental illness? Would people have weaponized my disorder if it had been something physical? I don't think so.

Yes, mental illness can affect behaviour, but I always say, "As long as someone is actively working on their stuff, I'm gonna be by their side as much as I can." And we tend to do that with other illnesses, just not with mental health.

My therapist and I use two major metaphors. One of them is the symbol of the dragon, which refers to the part of my disorder that was developed to protect me from others in situations of danger. A fire name and a fire mythological creature. And I realised I wasn't a damsel in distress guarded by a dragon that had to be slayed; I was the dragon itself, powerful, capable, terrified and terrifying, doing the best I could when confronted by random

knights trying to slay me in my own land. I looked at it with the eyes I use to look at all living creatures, trying to find beauty in their twists and cavities, and I've found some peace there.
I don't pray to the Goddess anymore for the pain to end. I barely pray anymore. My prayers are actions and my fire is not me chanting to a metaphor or candle wick – it is me handling the electricity impulses inside my nervous system, celebrating the wholeness of who I am: To some half monster, half human. I'm not afraid of monsters anymore, I'm afraid of those who create them. I don't "lick my wounds," I work to close my wounds, even if the scars limit my movements – but I don't let the infection spread. We learn so much of this in paganism, and in priestess training, yet it's not wisdom when these mantras are just repeated words in ritual context, or when they become justification for our actions. Goddess is pain too... but be responsible for yourself and don't use Goddess to hide the reason you don't work on what hurts.

Some of our brains will forever be marked by that fire, leaving scars like the ones lightning leave on the skin when striking a human – that, despite all odds, miraculously survives – scars forever invisible, eternally crippling, horribly beautiful. Who would I be without these scars? How would things have turned out? What could have been my full potential? These are questions without answers, leading to the frustration of the "what if," the untrue notion of the fake wholeness, the unreachable purity.

Last week, one of my drama teachers said that hurt people are special people, that our pain has made us unique. Fuck that, no! I don't want to be special, brave, resilient, strong... I want to be okay, I want peace, I want satisfaction, stability, I want a full life.

Let's stop romanticising being sick. The traits we try to hide as mystical abilities are mostly consequences of our pain. Yes, they can be used for good – but we have to recognise them as the mundane, sad thing that they are, instead of masking them like a gift from Goddess. Only then can we truly see Her – and the purpose we have in this world. You're never going to put your "empath abilities" to good use if you don't acknowledge that they might have come from your need to assess the situation to be safe – you're always going to endlessly project. What's wrong with the "mundane"? Isn't that Goddess, too? Doesn't that make it automatically sacred? Why the use of fancy names? Yes, I was scared, I learned to read people well. I can empathise with emotions now as a consequence of that. Let's stop being so self-conscious.

I was ashamed of my name in the same way I've come to be ashamed of the neurodivergence that resulted from the trauma some people inflicted on me – Something I had nothing to do with.

I wanted a mainlander name – a more common name – in the same way I've longed for (and wondered what it's like) to have a healed and "normal" brain. No, I'm not guilty for my trauma and its consequences, but I'm responsible for it now. And in the same fashion that I've come to love my name – despite its heavy meaning and how much it burns – I'm starting to maybe not love (but feel empathy and compassion for) that fiery monster made of electricity and fire... those paths of synapse that were birthed to protect me.

I told my therapist I didn't know what it was like to not have a neurodivergent brain. She said "No, but you know what it's like to be human." And I don't fight it anymore, I don't want to kill it or fix it – there's nothing wrong that needs "healing" or mending. I see it, I accept it, and I work with it, with *her*, with me. I'm whole as I am, chronically ill or not.

# Resting in Your Blue Shoes

Barbara O'Meara

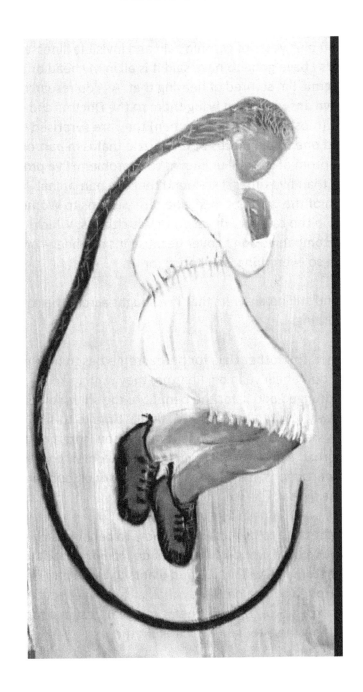

# Goddess Medicine, In Spite of Patriarchy

## Betsy Long

It's been 30 plus years of chronic pain and invisible illnesses that the Doctors I have gone to have said it is all in my head or that I am an enigma. I'm so tired of hearing that. As I do research and find my own answers, then bring them to the Doctors and specialists (mostly men, a few women) they are surprised that I have found one of the pieces of the puzzle that is in part only a direct symptom of the still unknown core problem. I've proven that more than five times; I've found that the patriarchal foundation of the world of medicine rarely listens to Women and puts them in the category of second-class citizens. Which insurance companies don't cover because it's not been coded in the system so everything is full price for us.

30 years and still no answers that I've sought across the country and yet nothing.

I have turned to Mother Gaia for herbal remedies to help my illnesses. I don't believe in big Pharma; they wish to keep everyone drugged and ill for the benefit of the shareholders. This is not the way to bring back our health. It's time to turn to our Goddesses, nature and heal ourselves as did our foremothers. It's time to learn. It's time to teach our younger women how to make tinctures, decoctions, herbal medicines to carry on our lines through the ages.

I've taken the time to take courses in how to become an herbalist in healing. I've used wonderful teas made from tree bark to soothe the stomach, wild herbs and plants to make painkillers. Walking through nature has always had a calming effect and a wondrous experience for me. It helps me heal, rest and forage medicinals that I use to help myself and others.

There is a long way to go.

Goddesses came into my life to help me heal in many ways. From the pain of a bad marriage and injuries I incurred from that, to the pain of my invisible illnesses. First it was Hecate to bring me back to life and help me realize I am not a helpless woman. I am Strong. I am FIERCE! I can heal myself! Then came the RAGE! Medusa to take back not only my life but my health and healing.

I look back on my life and The Goddesses have always been with me. The first time I realized this I was 11 in church. I started asking questions that the Patriarchal people of God did not like. I questioned how God made life without a woman. It was then that I left the church of the patriarchy behind. Yes, at a very early age I knew this wasn't truth. I had to find my way with Our Goddess.

I've been walking that path of Goddess and witchcraft/ paganism/ Shamanism ever since. The healing truth that I find is, Mama Gaia is our medicine and the only way back to her is to delve deeply into nature to find what we need individually to find our answers, to help each other heal their pain and illness. Look to the native cultures, Women's circles, Medicine women, through medicines of our ancestors and we will then thrive again as Women.

# Prayer Before the Rise of Goddess

Betsy Long

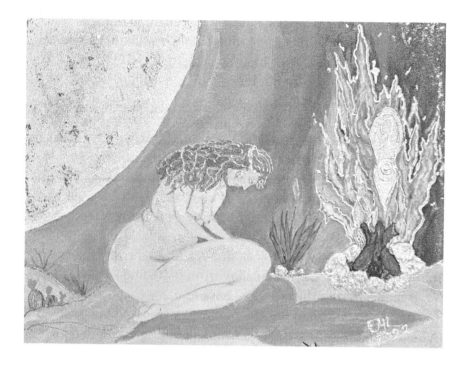

# Goddess and My Periods

Victoria Louise Lapping

The Goddess whispered to me softly
She told me to nurture my womb, to embrace my bleeds and all
that this would bring
Be gentle to myself, especially when bleeding, time to rest. Relax.
Go deep within and recover.
I did not listen.
How could I?!
Rest? Relax?
I had school to do, exams.
How could I just rest?
A struggle.
My energy dip was so low that every time I bled I would faint.
Every month, in hospital.
The Goddess softly told me, I need to nurture my womb.
 I was exerting myself doing too much.
My bleeds were time to withdraw.
Be still.
Patient.
I ignored her soft voice again.
How could I?
I had work, I had bills to pay, money and education to pursue.
You cannot rest not in this patriarchal society.
A woman has to keep going, never stop.
'No time' to stay still
A woman was only fit for society if she could multitask.
Dance her period away (in white pants no less) or so they say.
I grew worse.
High levels of stress causing chronic pain.
Too intense. Too heavy.
My hormones too large.
Every month getting more and more tests. Years of tests.
Finally diagnosed.

Endometriosis.
The Goddess now begged me to listen.
'Please nurture your womb.
Your bleeds are sacred.
If you rest, you will heal.
Connect with the divine feminine, she rests in you.
I rest in you. Embrace your bleeds. Rest my child.
Your society is not the way you are meant to live during a period.
You're meant to withdraw, rest, relax, be still during this time.
You were born for much greater things but no one was born to
multitask that is a repressive patriarchal construct.
Not the way of the Goddess. Please listen to your womb.'
I listened but I could not embrace, I was too ashamed, too full of
resentment, pain and annoyance and also grief for my body.
I let the Western medicine zap out hormone tissue.
I plucked up, masked up and removed my periods altogether
with a coil.
I removed the cause, removed my connection. Neglected my
womb.
I heard the Goddess whisper, I could not make out Her words,
was she crying?
She stopped.
No longer could I hear the Goddess, I had ignored Her for
too long.
Periods, not for everyone.
She surely could see the pain it was causing.
I was alone.
No bleeds
no Goddess
She left me be
just like I wanted.
For years I could not feel my connection, at first it was great.
No blood, no pain. No periods.
I loved it
but feeling of missing 'something' hit me, I felt disconnected.

I noticed a pattern – more medical professionals, more tests, more diagnosis
fibromyalgia, great, 'give her drugs'
chronic pain and fatigue 'give her the drugs'
IBS, perfect exactly what I need, 'give her more drugs'
chronic migraines and headaches worsening
just keeps coming, 'more drugs'
almost got a handle on it, then, buckled under pain
no help just the plaster to go over my deep bleeding wound.
Hide the problems with temporary fixes, mental health,
you guessed it – 'more drugs!' Drugs that make you a zombie.
Take away what makes me, me.
Enough.
No more feeling nothing. Being numb. Enough of medications and temporary fixes for long-term problems.
Enough of the side-effects and yet, more tablets, to counteract those tablets.
Enough.
I needed my connection back.
I needed to find me.
Remove the poisons.
The temporary fixes.
This final step. Remove the coil. This plastic object had given me fake hormones, cutting me off.
Get my period back.
At first I did not realise She was speaking but then Her voice became clearer.
I cried with relief.
I asked for forgiveness.
She whispered there is nothing to forgive.
I asked why, why I had to suffer.
I was upset, hurt, angry, mad, confused.
She told me I had to learn how to embrace my bleeds. Embrace my womb. I had not trusted my body enough, learn to heal, to grow, to nurture me.
I had been given all that I could have handled.

My choice was not a wrong choice, it is easy to get swept away, to hide the problem, to mask it, to run from it.

Periods are not nurtured. No one teaches you how to embrace they teach you how to hide the cramps, to keep going, keep moving, dancing, working.

How to pretend you are okay and never talk of your periods.

They remove, cut up, plug up, rip out, mask it. Silencing you.

Listen.

Embrace.

Embraced my period, a time to withdraw from the society and go within.

Rest. Relax.

I listened to the Goddess.

At least for a while.

Until I was diagnosed with 12 cm fibroid tumour growing in my uterus.

Worse now, extreme mood swings, food intolerances, excruciating pain.

I tried to tell the gynaecologist I did not want the temporary fixes.

I got scared.

They were good at convincing me, telling me the coil was my only option was my fault it was growing.

If I had the coil in, I would not have gotten this tumour.

My past trauma had created it and I had let it happen by taking out the coil.

If I just kept the coil in, it would not have grown. Symptoms would not be happening.

Blame.

Shame

Guilt

No options.

I asked the Goddess for guidance.

She told me to listen to my body.

I tried.

I really, really tried.

I felt my only option was to listen to the professionals.

Did it help?

No!

My moods got worse, anxiety heightened.

Spiritual awakenings began to occur. Questioning life, the goddess, the universe.

Strange.

That had never happened before.

Anxiety

Fear.

Uncontrollable, fear consumed me.

Like never before, strangled and suffocated me.

Anxiety filled my lungs.

A trip back to Gynaecology, told me it was definitely not the coil.

'Just my mental health.'

'Just my chronic pain.'

'Just to my stress, my trauma brain, my chronic pain,' excuse after excuse.

When I asked why I was bleeding still every single day she told me she had to put a cheaper brand of the coil in me as NHS cut on costs, so this one has more side effects.

'Get used to it.' They do not know the full side effects of this coil yet, I am their guinea pig.

My heart palpitations couldn't be due to the coil, it was 'just me'. Just my anxiety she said.

She told me that some women do get panic/palpitations however, and a lot more side effects with this new coil.

She could not see her own contradictions.

My partner asked her how long it would take the coil to shrink my fibroids.

'No' she laughed, 'whoever told you that?!?'

'This won't do anything for fibroids, just possibly stop it from growing, maybe, not sure, no proof that it helps but it 'might'.

But she was the one who told us it would shrink if I got the coil back in!

Deniability.

'Not her'.

We left, baffled, puzzled, confused.

I was angry
Over the next couple of weeks, I went deep within myself.
Listening.
Meditating.
Connecting.
My body wanted the coil out!
I waited to ensure it was a definite good idea.
I waited too long.
Questioning myself.
Anxiety crippling, debilitating.
'Get me out!'
A phone call to the best gynaecology department in my area, a
trip to E&E, six hours later, my coil finally out.
A brief moment of a doctor not finding coil.
New doctor questioned me. Was I definitely sure I wanted it out?
These 'hormones' could just be me? My programming?
My anxiety due to chronic illnesses and trauma.
Lots of 'are you sure' later finally... Out!
Instant she pulled it out, I felt I could breathe.
My stomach, my womb, my uterus.
Lighter.
Anxiety now lowered.
Yes, still high as I was in a hospital and covid was still a huge thing
at this point.
But felt more relaxed, more myself.
Huge relief! Smiled.
Car ride home I felt – just wonderful!
My partner noticed the change.
She had sensed, my nervous energy, the anxiety all of this time.
She felt a huge shift in me. My energy changed, more me.
She felt like I could finally breathe, and so did I.
Now this did not stop my fibroid. Did nothing for it either way
apparently.
But now?
Now I am working on it.
I am embracing my bleeds.

Still early days and I have a long way to go to fully connect in. Ten years of lost time to make up for.

And still trying to fix all my other pains, my periods, my body, my mental health.

Trying to meditate.

The Goddess patiently sitting by my side.

I am learning to heal my body.

My womb.

My pain.

My mind.

Only treatment options I have been offered are again temporary solutions.

No thanks!

I also have an inhospitable womb, so even if I want to, I could not/cannot carry a child in me.

It is too tilted, leaning against my IBS riddled bowels, too close to things, pressing on my spine – which may explain my bulging disc in lower back in my excruciating sciatica. When I questioned doctors they just laughed.

Some say it would be easier to rid myself of my womb entirely as, 'I do not need it', it 'cannot be used'.

One doctor said I am still too young to still have time to have babies, when I pointed out I can't she scrolled through my notes and said that with my partner and I both being women, she sees my point as two women cannot have children together.

The nurse quickly pointed out my wife could try carrying the child as an excuse for the doctor's homosexual ignorance.

The doctor was very confused why two women would want to have a child together?!

Other doctors tell me to remove my womb as I do not need it, there is no use for it.

Which can cause a lot more future problems than it is worth like dementia

I am okay, more than ok, with not been able to carry a child.

It is not in the cards for me.

But I do not want to take out my womb, just because of fibroids.

There are herbal teas, remedies and meditations/mindfulness practices I can do to naturally heal myself.
I now enjoy the winter rest of my bleeds.
My power in the magic of my moon blood.
I am learning and healing the anxiety of my autumn (premenstrual)
Embellishing my Power of spring and summer.
A womb is not only a place you can give life to babies.
It is my sacred femininity.
A place I can birth ideas.
Projects and creations.
Come into my power of my sacred femininity.
We each have this power within us (even if you have to get a hysterectomy or don't bleed).
We can each tap into the power of our sacred centre.
Asking for guidance
Inspiration to birth ideas and creations
All we have to do is listen.
The Goddess is patiently sitting by my side.
I am learning to heal my body.
My womb.
My pain.
My mind.
So now the Goddess and I use visualisation to strengthen my life.
I am learning the balance of this patriarchal society and the sacred femininity.
The Eastern and Western medicine.
To connect with nature.
To my power within.
To my periods.
To the Goddess.
But most importantly... To connect with me.
Can you hear her whispering?
She is calling to you.

# *Cocooning*

## Barbara O'Meara

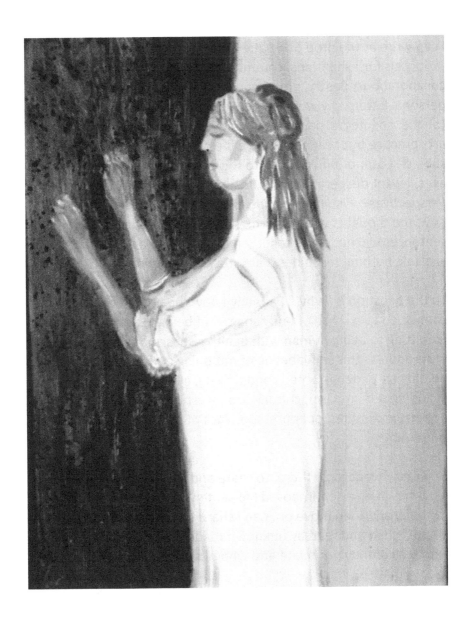

# I Need to Grieve for my Body and Move on

### Barbara O'Meara

I can write at the drop of a hat – artist's statements, creative proposals for exhibitions, community art workshops, artistic collaborations, poetry, prose, spoken word songs, rhymes, personal letters, my words are always there on the tip of my tongue, an integral part of my creative being alongside my visual arts practice but I cannot 'for the life of me' find the words for this subject. I cannot find a way into this piece. I have been trying for ages, I want desperately to write about my experiences of *Pain Perspectives – Finding Meaning in the Fire* but there is no word flow, the thoughts will not form, ideas are not generating, the sentences will not string together, I cannot find an angle, the page is blank, nothing resonates. I am stuck! I am never stuck!

So the question is 'Why'? I already know the answer and it is connected to a sense of body shame, of being less than perfect, of admitting to being human with health issues and flaws. So now I must address this self-labeling of not being a perfect woman. I am holding on to deep-rooted conditioning, a lifetime of criticism including self-criticism, cultural brainwashing, absorbing unsafe notions and values, peer pressure, lack of confidence and my own self-doubt.

Do I really want to go there, to share and to bare my soul about what has been a self-imposed life sentence? I need to grieve for my body and then move on. Can I share this in a book which will be published and read by unknown readers who do not know me, who may or may not relate and who may judge me? Yes I can.

Why? Because now is the right time, and this is the right place, a women's creative space where I will be among other women who are confronting their own pain perspectives. I must address my body image issues once and for all now, a daunting task because it is so personal to me, about me, and about my deepest pain. During the past year of my life everything has changed drastically. I have been on an extremely physical healing journey which I have survived and this has finally allowed me to put the past into perspective. That was then and this is now the perfect time to acknowledge, allow, accept, grieve and release in order to move forward.

It is difficult to revisit the words I wrote on this subject many months ago and not least because how I felt then and what I wrote is no longer relevant. I am here, I am alive. Admittedly I have not yet fully healed so writing this piece is the closure I need.

I am someone who likes to move forward; even after taking a wrong turn while driving I cannot turn back – I must go on and trust I will find a way to arrive at the correct destination. I have always had the precious ability to see and honor the divine essence of beauty in all women yet I cannot see this in myself. I still have these un-dealt with feelings of loss for the woman I used to be. As a feminist, a women's rights arts activist, an educator with a focus on empowering other women, I have often wondered why I have not honored and accepted my own body. As a young woman I was diagnosed with an auto immune disease which affected my physical appearance. My body changed; this was the very least of my health issues but it seemed to have affected me in the most damaging way.

I was and still am a so called 'normal' shape, just more abundant, more Goddess-like but this awareness did not ease my body shame. Positive mental attitude, gratitude, cultivating deep inner beauty and valuing of characteristics like empathy and integrity were all part of my strategy to cope. As an artist I had a deep appreciation for the beauty of the human body and perhaps because of this and early childhood conditioning, an impossible striving for perfection (even though I am well aware that there is no such thing). As a young woman I had this unattainable desire for flawlessness which seems so ridiculous now, as an older woman.

Since my healing journey I am in a different head space. I have looked back at health issues, my denial, my pain, my frustration; I have faced what I could not let go of for the longest time, the loss of my old self and my perceived identity. Coming to a new phase of my life as I move toward my Crone years, I do not have the time or the energy to invest in any more resentment toward the unfairness of ill health or the injustice of managing a chronic disease. Performing a farewell ritual for my past with fitting funerary burial rights I am moving on. Now positioning myself with a new approach to self-appreciation, with more kindness and self-care, developing and nurturing non-judgmental relationships and interactions with others and indeed with myself, I know that my advancing years have given me a certain amount of freedom over a regretful past body image.

Communicating trustfully with other women has also been a wonderful way to open up and to realize that every woman has body issues. For many years I sat in women's circles at sacred ceremonies and gatherings where there is almost always the protection of sisterhood that has allowed me to safely initiate the healing process for my body shame.

My own daughters are strong, kind, sensitive, assertive and self-confident, and raising them with body awareness that has only ever been a topic of positive reinforcement, they have rarely felt judged, self-conscious, or lesser than what they are – powerful young women with healthy, functioning, active bodies, who have taken up space in their physical beings and in the world. They are ordinary yet extraordinary young women, non-judgmental of other women, they see the uniqueness of all women and they see me, their mother, with the vision of unconditional love. I have wanted to "be normal', to "look average", to "fit in" for myself and for them for the whole of my mothering life and now I realize that this has never mattered to them, that they never saw me as I viewed myself. I am so accepting towards others yet I have not accepted myself.

Now I need to honor the Goddess within me. As a mother I am loving, present, protective and supportive... and I finally realize that all these things that I have been for my daughters, I have not been for myself.

And so finally I say 'STOP'.... no more discussion, enough is enough... I will not allow my body to define me as a woman divine. I now understand that self-intervention is the key to prevention of shame and suffering and that treasuring my feminine essence is the best possible way to self-empowerment. I embrace my womanhood with conscious pure self-love as I adorn my body with glorious textiles and jewels. My healing journey has been the greatest incentive to propel myself forward into loving all that I am. It has given me permission to not compartmentalize my trauma and pain, to not bury it deeply and hold it in my body where it may fester and stay alive. The self-inflicted shame I often considered to be a vanity, I now name it, I own it, I purge it and I release it. In the past I would have considered these words to be a bit of a pity party, typically having little self-compassion but I no longer want or need to live with this detrimental self-judgment. I am a real imperfect woman allowing only openness and honesty. I acknowledge with acceptance and with much appreciation, my one precious life in the hope of growing old both gracefully and disgracefully. I cherish all women supporting women, empathically embracing you all. I wish you all the strength to courageously stand in your own healing power so that you may not only survive but may also thrive.

# *Self-Portrait*

Barbara O'Meara

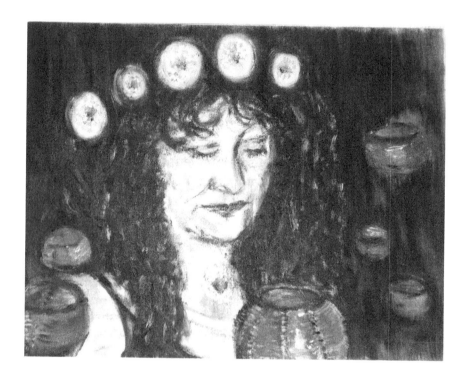

# The Weight of My Mother's Trauma

Victoria Earle

This pain I bear, this ache that nags and pulls me down day after day, is it mine or hers?

Does this searing, burning fatigue start with me or my mother? I only know it is worse when I am with her: I never feel so old as when I enter her house.

A mother who received no mothering herself. A mother whose own mother died in labour.

This bone-leaching ache that keeps me stuck, that neither doctor nor naturopath can name. Burn-out, Depression, Chronic Fatigue, Polymyalgia, Fibromyalgia are labels but not names.

I need a name for this dream thief. I need to trace it to the source.

I need to track it to the centre of the forest. I need to put out the fire, not just cough up the smoke.

I ask Her to guide me: the Great Dark Mother who holds me as I toss and turn through fretful, ear-ringing nights. I pray to Her who knows, I trust She will be there when I am ready.

Then one night my octogenarian mother tells her daughter this: that my father hit her, that he knocked her to the ground, that he shot her (and missed), that she fled to the neighbours, that he overdosed, that his family gaslit her, that he broke into her home and stole her jewellery.

And my judgement of her falls away. I no longer see a weak and needy woman. I see someone who used all her strength to leave my father. A woman who has carried this inside her for fifty years. I understand everything and nothing.

And I sleep the deepest sleep. And the next day the pain is less, and the day after that, and the day after that.

As it slowly ebbs away, I name my pain *The Weight of my Mother's Trauma.*

I see myself in the centre of the forest. I've found the fire. I've put it out. And next to it I build a new one from the embers, made with kindness, compassion and gratitude.

I light it with my dreams, dreams that seemed impossible until now.

And I feel Her watching over me, blessing it. I sense my mother and grandmother beside me.

And I name this new fire *The Healing of the Mother Line.*

# *Fire Dancer*
## Kat Shaw

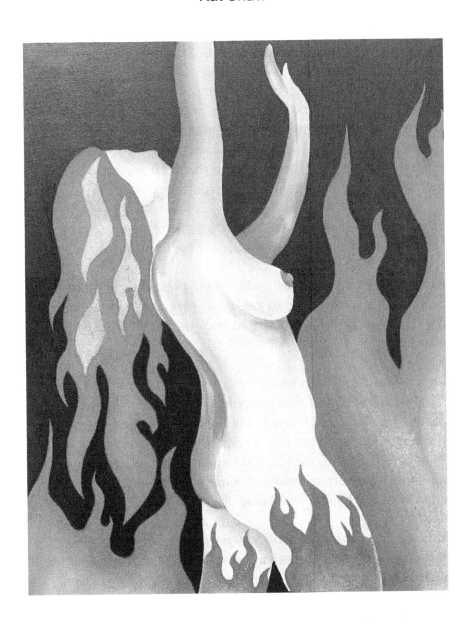

# Many Forms of Pain and A Little Perspective

Deborah A. Meyerriecks

Pain comes in so many different forms. Sometimes it's sudden as with a major injury that heals but never stops hurting entirely. Other times it's a gradual onset of symptoms that accumulate and take over to the point where one can't remember what started the chain reaction. Some of us have mental or emotional pain that was taken less seriously because it wasn't medical or trauma-related. When pain becomes old and chronic it generally invites mental and emotional pain in for the duration.

Physical, Emotional, Mental, Spiritual. Pain, healing, and growth can generally fall into one or more of these four categories.

Pain had been a part of my life for so long that the absence of it became unsettling. I used to joke (in all seriousness) that pain let me know I was still alive. I used to also say that I'd sleep when I was dead.

I remember when I was very young, trying to talk with my mother, my grandparents, and them responding to me completely out of context to what I was trying to tell them, *what I needed to tell them.* I remember when that turned into getting no response at all or being told they didn't want to hear it (or me.) It wasn't all the time. It was often enough to leave a lasting imprint on my emotional and mental well-being. No one wanted to hear me.

This was thoroughly reinforced by my grandfather proclaiming that children should be seen and not heard. Often. And a father who didn't understand the words *no... stop... why I was crying...* or why disdain or quiet anger replaced my tears whenever I needed to be with him.

I learned to sit on the sidelines and be quiet. To not share my thoughts unless asked, and even then, to limit what I said. I learned not to want or need anything. I learned that the loneliest place to be is often surrounded by people who claim to love you but seemingly do not like you.

As an older child who was permitted to go out and wander alone, I would talk. The voice in my head kept me company. I thought I was talking to myself. I would say hello to the trees and imagine I saw them wave hello to me as I approached. I'd whisper my secrets to the breeze and the night winds and believe I could hear voices whispering back that they heard, understood, and most of all, believed me. I loved to be near and in the water. Baths, lakes, ocean, rain... all of it. I wasn't very fond of the bright sun because it made my eyes hurt and more than that, it made it difficult to hide when you felt like there was a spotlight on you.

I learned to climb trees on my own. I loved the feeling of being isolated up in the air while still grounded through the tree trunk to the earth. I started to crave the feeling of being surrounded by branches and leaves. I never was concerned with falling. I felt supported. As I would lay back on a perfectly angled branch and rest, I not only hugged the tree, but the tree hugged back.

I had developed similar relationships with all the elements. While the Sun was blinding, sometimes it was soft. Sunrise and sunset remain my favorite times of day. Fire is another relationship. Fire spoke to me and danced for me. Water surrounded, supported, and held me. Water also tuned out the rest of the world. I was never lonely while in nature.

I don't remember what age I was when my father started to sexually abuse me. I just don't remember a time when he didn't. Chronic headaches and belly aches were normal, just as it was normal for those complaints to be ignored and then seemingly unheard. What I was taught is that my own pain or discomfort was inconsequential. What I learned was to just live with it. I was taught to downplay how much things bothered me or hurt and to gaslight myself that it probably wasn't as bad as I thought it was. Especially when it came to having to spend visitation weekends or weeks with my father.

He was attentive during those visits. Asking how school was and what I wanted to eat for breakfast or dinner. I learned that attention meant discomfort or pain. I learned to associate admitting that I wanted anything with certain prices that would need to be paid. I also learned how to disassociate and astral project. If I simply refused to be present for, or participate in, the moments of pain, I didn't have to feel them. My body would endure but I wouldn't remember. I created a safe place that I now recognize as sacred space that I could escape to whenever reality was too hard or painful to remain present in.

During my astral travels, I would talk no longer with myself as the voice in my head became clearly not my own. Goddess distracted me and comforted me. She taught me many things that I still incorporate in my personal practice as witch, healer, and priestess.

Those wounds eventually healed but they left scars that can throb and ache when poked or irritated.

During the course of a career dedicated to helping others, I would have a few accidents. Broken ankles, sprained knees, strained shoulders. The pain was never as bad for me as I was told it should have felt. Pain was something I always carried within me. Not quite knowing how to let it go. The last time I got hurt at work, I sustained a permanent fracture in one ankle and 6 vertebral fractures of my lower spine. The pain of the spinal spasms was at times unbearable. I felt like I was drowning in it. On the pain scale, a 10 is the worst pain you have ever felt in your life. I was at a 10+.

A month into my slow recovery, I received a text asking what color candle they should use for that night's Full Moon. Something took over and I started to compose the longest email I ever wrote. Starting with the magickal focus of each phase of the moon and detailing magical color correspondence and everything else I could think of. Only thing is, I wasn't thinking. I felt hijacked in a good way. I felt full and nurtured from within. The voice in my head had taken over and was pouring information and direction though my fingers on the keyboard. I vaguely remember feeling like I wanted to tell them to look it up and leave me alone, oh and by the way, the current moon phase was new. Goddess stepped in and gave me something to give them to use for reference and then gave me the first deep and restful sleep I'd had since my accident.

It would be a long year of fighting with doctors to get physical therapy until one doctor very early in my recovery was allowed to give me (because worker's comp was paying the bills). This one doctor gave me a series of gentle movements that I could do at home and then let me know he couldn't help me any further.

Left with an intolerance or allergy to most pain medication and no one to guide my physical rehab, I asked the voice inside my head for help. Help came again. Sometimes like a drill sergeant ordering me to move when I could, ordering me to rest when I felt like I could do more. And simply saying "I know," acknowledging me when I cried in pain and frustration.

While feeling absolutely broken and incapable of ever being useful or of service again; when the pain and heartbreak from old, original scars told me that people could only want me when I'm useful and won't want me now that I can't be, the voice told me I was wrong. When I had trouble believing it and tried to silence my cries from emotional and physical pain that I knew would always be there, She opened my eyes to see my (then) partner and my no longer young children (my Dynamic Duo) who chose to stay close and take care of each other and of me when I couldn't take care of them or myself.

When I still felt the need to be of service to feel self-worth, the voice inside my head whispered ideas and words that flowed through my fingers and keyboard onto the screen. A new lesson in WitchCraft or a new guide for working with Moon phases and Solar stations around the Wheel of the Year flowed each week to make 52 lessons I would email to a small list of people who had been asking for more after they received the first lesson. 13 New Moon, 13 Full Moon, 8 for the first day of each new season, and 18 progressive lessons that gave the foundation to start one's own personal right path in the Craft.

And to keep me moving, the automatic writing would suddenly disconnect. Left feeling a little off for a few moments, I would get up and slowly wander in circles trying to decide what I needed in that moment. Movement. That's what I needed. And almost always, nourishment. Tea is still almost always the answer. It's just that these days, I have to remain caffeine free.

When I was 6 years into my healing process with better mobility but still had chronic pain and the fatigue that came with it, I had a sudden feeling of extreme exhaustion. Nothing hurt and I just wanted to go back to bed and lie down. The voice inside my head, my Goddess, wouldn't let me. Feeling winded and not able to catch my breath, mild confusion about things such as whether I'd had anything to drink yet that day or if I left my teacup and water glass on the counter from the night before... Several voices were now in my head, one telling me I needed a 12-lead EKG, another telling me I needed to go to the ER now, another yelling at me to *under no circumstance* was I to drive myself!!! My Dynamic Duo were upstairs, my now ex (who had remained my close friend) walked in the front door unexpectedly as I was just standing there processing. When he asked me if I was ok and I admitted that I didn't know, he ordered me to get into his car and called upstairs to my son and daughter that he was taking me around the block to the hospital.

Seriously, for the first time in a very long time, nothing hurt. And I was so exhausted. I remembered all the times I ever said that pain is what reminds me I'm still alive and that I would sleep when I was dead. Maybe, I thought to myself, I was dying. "Not if we can help it. Get in his car, now." I heard.

Not from anyone in the house but from the voice inside my head. From my Goddess.

Minutes later I was in the ER and being prepared for transfer by EMS to the local Cardiac Cath Lab. I was having a massive heart attack known as an Acute Myocardial Infarction or AMI. I read my own 12-lead EKG when the ER doctor showed it to me. I was having a triple STEMI, and ST (part of the EKG wave pattern) Elevated MI (Myocardial Infarction.)

I was on the phone to my Dynamic Duo from the back of an ambulance with a medic who remembered me from my younger days when I was an EMT in Coney Island, NYC. The biggest concern for all of us was my known allergies to pain meds.

In the Cath Lab, a nurse was assigned to stay near me where we could talk. She let me know everything they were doing and what they were giving me to keep me comfortable and calm. She made it very clear to the cardiac surgeon that he could not give me the usual morphine or valium or anything else. The surgeon told me he wouldn't as long as I remained still. I assured him I would. I knew what was coming. He needed to cut deep enough into my inner thigh near the groin in order to gain access to my femoral artery. Then he needed to puncture it and thread a catheter into it, then thread it up into my heart.

This was going to hurt. A lot. I opened myself and called out to my Goddess. I didn't ask to have my pain taken away or to not feel it. I said to Her that I knew She knew I had this, but if She could hold me still while I had this procedure I would be grateful.

I felt a heavy weight over my whole body as if someone were laying on top of me and we had a weighted blanket over the both of us. I felt warm breath on my left cheek. I felt my own tear on my face as the surgeon cut into me. I remained absolutely still. Everything went well and soon I was resting in recovery and preparing to go home the next morning.

New pain will come and hopefully go. Some pains have remained with me since I was a child. Through them all, I know I have never truly been alone. Goddess has always been with me. I've learned to do what I can and rest before I need to. I don't always remember to do that for myself. When I over-do, I don't have the choice and the following several days were forced rest and recovery days.

In recent years, I have been working on those Soul-deep Shadow wounds and scars. I am learning how to recognize what I need and ask for it – from myself and from those who love me completely. The ones who only want me to take good care of myself and continue to let them in. The ones who will always hear me, even when I'm not using my words.

I have found perspective through my pain and through the whole process, Goddess has been with me, cradling me, holding my hand, and cheering for me as I climb high and receive the bliss and joy I once found so elusive and believed would always be out of my reach.

# *Scarred*
## Kat Shaw

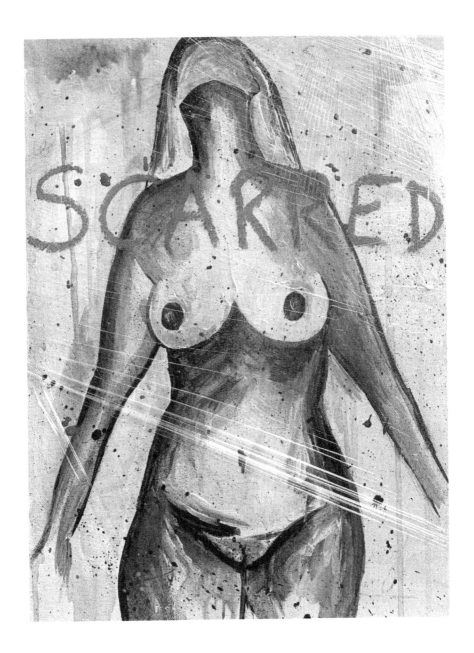

# Torch Bearing Goddesses

### Deborah A. Meyerriecks

Goddess on the Battlefield
Fighting by my side
Goddess of Compassion
Hold me as I heal
Goddess of Strength
Guide me as I fight
Goddess of Love
Bear witness to my release

Pain, Battle, Surrender, Repeat

Some days progress
Some nights retreat

Pain, Battle, Surrender, Recoup

Remembering what once could easily be done
Finding acceptance in what limitations persist
Working toward what may be done again

Pain, Battle, Surrender, Revise

Lost who was and discover who is
Fire burns the chaff away and tempers the gold within
Leaving seen and unseen scars
Goddess passes Her torch into my hand

Pain, Battle, Surrender, Realize

Isolated and feeling alone
Yet filled and enveloped by Goddess
Holding the torch in the dark
So others who needn't find their way alone
May carry the torch further for others

Pain, Battle, Surrender, Release

# *Brigid's Flame*

## Barbara O'Meara

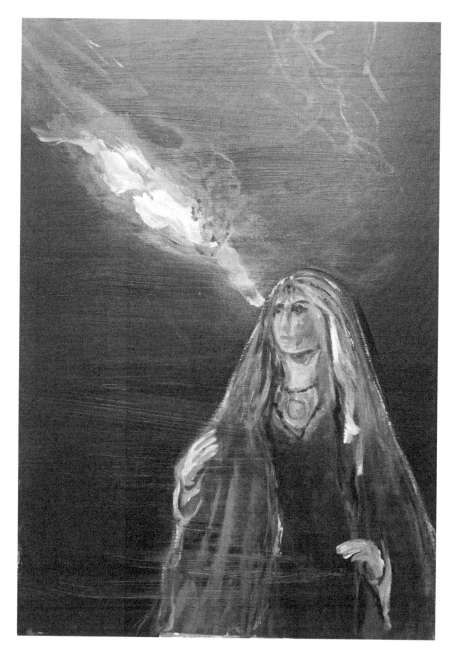

# Out of the Flames

Rebekah Myers

Women are in pain.
Why is this so?
What can we do to find release and healing?

Illness among women is on the rise.

In a recent study of nineteen different autoimmune illnesses, it was found that these impact ten percent of the population, with thirteen percent of women and seven percent of men being affected. A paper published in May of 2023 explores a rise in these nineteen autoimmune diseases from previous estimates, and examines evidence that factors other than genetic ones are likely involved (Dr Nathalie Conrad, Professor Iain McInnes, Professor Geraldine Cambridge, "Incidence, prevalence, and co-occurence of autoimmune disorders over time and by age, sex, and socioeconomic status: a population-based cohort study of 22 million individuals in the UK, May 5, 2023).

Cardiovascular disease and coronary artery disease are the number one cause of death for women in the United States and are often harder to diagnose than for men. Some in the medical profession suggest that this may be due to a lack of adequate acknowledgement and care from doctors, and from women being culturally and socially conditioned to put themselves last, and men being conditioned to put themselves first (Kavitha Chinnaiyan, M.D., Beaumont cardiologist, Beaumont Health System, 2023).

Recent studies find an increase in cervical cancer in women sixty-five and older, and an increase in pancreatic and breast cancers are on the rise among younger women (Brigham and Women's Hospital Communications September 8, 2022).

Emotional and mental illnesses are also prevalent as many women find that their health issues and experiences are minimized, gaslit, or used against them to discredit them by patriarchal figures in positions of power.

It may be that my own two autoimmune illnesses, and my daughter's endometriosis, CSF leaks, and pre-autoimmune symptoms were exacerbated, if not caused altogether by the conditions imposed by the social system of the patriarchy.

What is the patriarchy?

Patriarchal social systems glorify personal power and gain at all costs. The desecration and destruction of the earth and its waterways, flora and fauna, means nothing as long as it results in power and gain. These attitudes and acts cause inflammatory reactions in the earth itself and the delicate balance throughout the web of life is thrown out of kilter. Illness and pain are the outcome, and this imbalance makes its way within the web to human beings where it is manifest inside us as well.

Within a patriarchal social structure, women are often discouraged from achieving financial independence and instead are encouraged to remain within the confines of the family home, caring for the needs of the household, the children, and a male partner. Often, a man will earn more money than his wife or female partner, and this will cause an imbalance of power within the relationship. Believe it or not, there are still marital situations today where a woman is financially dependent on her husband or male partner and must ask his permission regarding even basic grocery items or the payment of utility bills. There are still partnerships today where women are being abused, either emotionally, verbally, financially, or physically. Why don't they leave? Because of their financial dependence. Often, it is more frightening to face full financial hardship than to continue enduring a familiar if damaging situation of abuse.

Although my own father was supportive and encouraged me to get my education and degree, my religious organization did not. It may be that despite my father's positive influence, the influence of my religious circle had a stronger impact upon my choices in the early years of my adulthood. Young girls are taught from a very early age in my religion's culture, to be stay-at-home mothers and to give up a career outside the home for one inside. Church leaders will recommend an education for women, but from the other side of their mouths state that after receiving one, it should be used to be a better mother.

If time reveals a marriage partner to be entrenched in patriarchal thought, or to be damaged by it in various aspects of his life, a financially dependent woman with dependent children can find herself in a devastating situation. To suffer prolonged abuse of any kind from a person you live closely with, and upon whom you are dependent, can have catastrophic effects on a woman's health, and on the health of her growing children as well over time. I believe that this is what happened to me, and to my children also.

A few years ago, a blood test revealed that I had Hashimoto's Disease, and about a year after that, I found myself at death's door from undiagnosed Addison's Disease/Primary Adrenal Insufficiency. Both of these are autoimmune diseases – the former is caused when one's own immune system attacks and destroys the thyroid gland, and the latter is caused when it attacks and destroys the adrenal glands. Both these glands produce hormones essential to life. Without the proper amounts, your body shuts down and you die. No doctor out of the many I visited, understood what was happening to me, and most told me to run along home and breathe deeply. In the eleventh hour, when I was in full-blown adrenal crisis, this condition was finally caught, and my life was saved, if never to be the same.

The strange and scary symptoms I experienced, the long sleepless nights filled with pain and fear, the dismissal from doctors, and the lack of caring or support from my partner were a crucible of fire within which I suffered greatly. There were times when my flesh burned and I was hot to the touch. There were times when it felt as if a ball of burning fire was passing through my body from the top of my head down and out through my feet.

It is a known medical fact that constant duress is harmful to the body. My former husband actually got a charge from upsetting me. It was fun for him to threaten me and to see my mounting distress. Many times, I did a good job of not reacting to him, but it always affected me adversely inside. This occurred on a regular basis for many years. Imagine the extra work my thyroid and adrenal glands had to do to support me, as stress surged throughout my system.

The thyroid and the adrenal glands are both a part of the body's endocrine system. Mine had to work overtime. Bobbi Parish, MA, says: "Narcissist abuse and trauma survivors are often diagnosed with chronic pain and autoimmune disorders because long-term exposure to cortisol and adrenaline (fight or flight chemicals) cause inflammation in our bodies. Inflammation causes pain, or worse, it causes our immune system to attack itself because it thinks the inflammation is caused by a disease it needs to eradicate."

Men who have been raised in the patriarchal social system are likewise inflamed. They become damaged and crippled by this, emotionally and psychologically. This is a system that teaches boys to be ashamed of feelings or actions of tenderness, empathy, compassion, or nurturing. This is a system that teaches boys to place girls and women at low value, to be suspicious of them, to blame them, to disrespect them. Men raised in a patriarchal social system often have a sense of entitlement. Simply by virtue of them being born male, they are taught to expect the women in their lives to serve, obey, and defer to them. These men are often unable to have meaningful relationships with women and can only relate to the feminine as objects designed for their pleasure, and under their control. Patriarchal societies often produce misogynistic men, and this misogyny springs from a deep distrust and fear. Often these men are aghast and will protest vehemently if this phenomenon is brought to their attention, but underneath this outward protestation, the ingrained destructive behaviors continue.

Two years after my chronic autoimmune illnesses were diagnosed, I began attending a local Red Tent circle. Many things about it were empowering to me, and as I researched and studied various aspects of women's spirituality, I realized that I had a desire to give and share within this large, worldwide community. I started facilitating my own women's spirituality circles and creating meaningful ritual and ceremony. I started writing about it. I created social media pages and groups dedicated to the edification, education, and empowerment of women and their brothers. All of this has been tremendously exciting, healing and fulfilling to me.

Where is the Goddess in all of this? Front and center. After years of only finding Her in folklore, fairy tales, mythology, and neo pagan movements, I now find Her in completeness everywhere. My path now is an eclectic mix of women's wisdom, earth and nature spirituality, cyclical living and intersectional feminism – all of which are elements of the Goddess way. My fiery furnace of physical and emotional pain, sorrow, fear, and devastation burned away the non-essential and left in its wake a clarity of understanding, wisdom, and the will to forge a new way.

Men and boys need their Mother just as much as girls and women do. All human beings need to develop what are traditionally known as feminine traits and masculine traits within themselves to achieve a state of balance and wholeness. Those traits traditionally known as feminine, that patriarchy has so devalued, must be understood to be necessary, and be embraced and developed. Patriarchal approaches to life on this planet need to be dismantled. These approaches have not served us well. They have made women sick and they have made Mother Earth sick.

But there is hope. While damage has been done, and essential things may have been lost along the way, healing, renewal, and a joyful creative energy is born from the pain of the past.

# *Taranaki*

## Stephanie Mines

The Texture of Oppression
In the bodies of the women who come to me for healing
I feel the texture of oppression:
Strings of coagulated holding back in musculature,
Poison pellets of self-rejection, inserted deeply into connective
tissue.
Taut tendons entwine bone like strangulation vines emitting
Venomous inflammation.
I touch the ectoderm of centuries of agony,
The mesoderm of shock, and
The braced membrane of endoderm, defiant and impenetrable.
Fluids meant to flow are backed up, filling
Avenues of expression with sediment, making them
Pathways of refusal.
Latched back doors to the heart long to swing open to the front,
To release the pent-up spontaneity that has been damned.
The time has come, my sisters,
To disbar the court that silences us from within.
The time has come to detoxify the texture of oppression
From our flesh, and
Come out from the eddy of repetitious restraint.
We can do this. We can irrigate with rivulets of permission,
With waves of validation and recognition, the
Brine of wisdom that is the song, the poem, the art of
The crone. Invoke, supplicate
She who dwells in our wombs, she who knows
How we give birth to ourselves.

Stephanie Mines, Copyright, 2023

# Pain and Patriarchy I

Claire Dorey

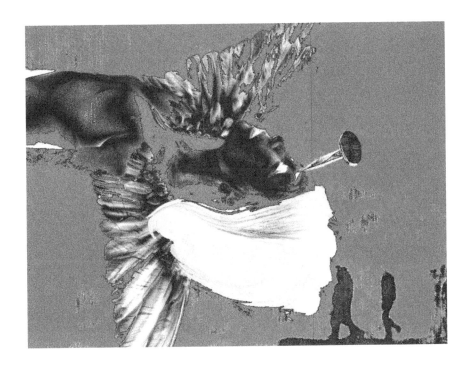

# Pain and Patriarchy II

Claire Dorey

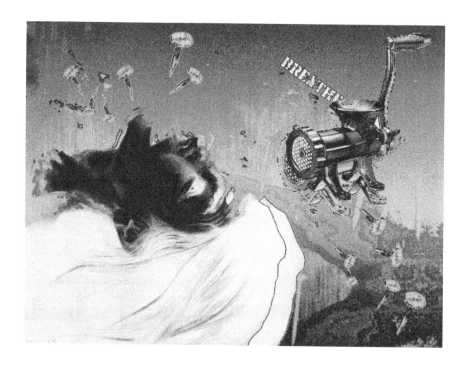

# Pain and Patriarchy III
Claire Dorey

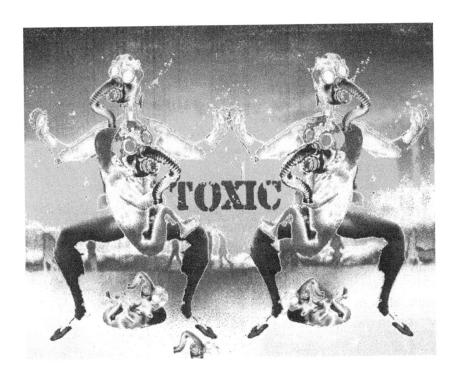

# If Pain Was A Labyrinth

Claire Dorey

If pain was a labyrinth
I'd meet you at the centre
I'd take you to that Minotaur
Because the story of chronic pain
Is best not faced alone

I believe there is a seed of patriarchal wounding lodged in the heart of every woman.

If pain was a woman, it would be half woman, half fish. Ophelia's glazed eyes staring skywards, waterlogged robes, pulling her down. Female pain is a Siren's sigh, a lament lingering in the mist that hangs above the sea. Sailors, drifting near the Otherworld where women rule, fear the Siren's sigh because deep in their souls, all men know they are protagonists in the tragicomedy of what man has done to woman.

On stage the tragic farce is still unfolding. Masked actor, manipulators accuse women of the demonic and the laughable! It's a nonsense, so puerile, it is unanswerable.

What if I told you that "Pain is your inheritance"?

We all carry an imprint of inherited pain. Traumatic pain is part of being female.

If you don't believe me, scroll through the fusty pages of time to see how scientists, philosophers and religious experts wrote, into official texts, how and why, woman is inferior. Organised religion condemned woman at her most vulnerable – giving birth. They told us the pain of childbirth was payback for the sin of being born female. We tolerated wagging fingers and outrageously callous lectures about Original Sin because we had no option, our survival depended on it.

Women drowned in this vindictive system. We became mute, co-dependent. Our authentic voice, the Siren's sigh, fled into the ocean with a hiss!

Back on land, their psychologists told us we were neurotic and hysterical. They told us we had penis envy and when they abused us, they said we were asking for it! Their words were like whips. We could no longer recognise ourselves.

I could go on...

If pain were a labyrinth it would rage like a whirlpool. A life going down the plughole. A seed resting in the heart poised to spiral into allergies and inflammation. Pain is a calcified stone. A state of numb. A cold slab. A dead-end corridor. The stone-cold passages of power. A maze of condescending comments and dead-end attitudes. A howl barrelling down the tunnels. Pain is a mask. The Minotaur is its metaphor. Pain is shame. Pain is lonely, exhausting, an all-consuming dish served icy cold. Pain is a destination. Familiar surroundings. Some pass through. Others inhabit it. Some of us drown in it.

If the labyrinth were menstrual cramps, it would be a hot mess of suffering. A form of paralysis. A dull thud of misery. The body crying out, month after month, begging us to notice that it is no use trying to fit into a system that is not kind to us.

You told us we were unclean. You cast us out. Banished us to the outhouse. Chucked a cloth over us. You told us we were offensive in our natural state. We absorbed this shame.

If pain were a river, it would be a river in a hurry. Water springs from a slit in the slate, high up in the foothills. Then it gathers momentum and barrels through the forest, shamanic drumming in full throttle, pummelling giant blocks of quartz into pebbles. An overlay of saintdom has been assigned to this river but we all know the Goddess of wild places lives here. Rather than slowing down as it nears the sea, this river speeds up, carving a jagged canyon in the slippery slate cliffs, before it descends to the ocean in a series of stepped waterfalls – and it is here that I slipped and fell into the torrent. I hurt my back. The pain makes me vulnerable. How can I survive this ruthless, dominator culture if I am not in pristine condition?

My sigh joins the collective Siren's sigh that flows down the river and out to sea as a tidal wave, landing on the shore of the Island Of Tears, populated by half women, half fish. It is here that water stores memory. Can we purge our pain by throwing our intention to heal into the ocean?

If pain were a chart, it would be graded from one to five, so an expert can categorise, capitalise or dismiss it. Give form to the formless. Why? Because they can't conceive of pain as an 'abstract'. How can you grade the generational trauma that women have experienced? It has played havoc with our nervous systems. We are all survivors of this suppressor regime where justice has always been stacked on the side of the perpetrator, the establishment and white male privilege. How do you grade the chronic pain of red alert when the receptors won't switch off?

We fell for the mis-sold myth of the white dress and waited for the black dress. You lured us into a life of domestic slavery, whilst our 'Fathers' sat in their carver chair at the head of the table, lording over Nourishment. Food became a power struggle, a lesson in hierarchy. No wonder we fed that Minotaur with self-loathing and eating disorders.

When we fought for our freedom, you made us stand in the dark and denied us a chair. Your tools of torture, to extract our 'confessions', became ever more creative, demonic, sadistic and sexualised: the Pricking Test; the Iron Maiden; the Swimming Test and the Ducking Stool.

You stoned us to death and buried us in the ground.

You burnt us alive.

I have to pause a moment, writing this is making me feel quite traumatised. This grotesque horror show seems so unbelievably fantastical but this story of what they did to us, is true!

When did the system abandon women? When did it decide to obliterate our skills and knowledge? When did it lose empathy for our sense of grief, loss and rejection? Abandonment is a raw, painful and traumatic experience. Who cast the first stone?

Patriarchy is psychological warfare for women. It got us on our knees, clutching our guts. We face it down every single day we poke our peachy toes out of the door.

If female pain was a shoe, it would be a stiletto, a precarious balance of objectified submission and weaponised sexuality.

Because the form of Natural Woman was never good enough, we wore crippling corsets and debilitating shoes, just to please you.

You told us we could dominate you if we strapped ourselves in leather and spikes and smashed you about a bit! You paid us to humiliate you for fun, in the same way you humiliated us for real. You turned the torture you subjected us to into 'play' and reduced us to whores!

If pain was a Minotaur, a contorted and twisted creature, it would be banished to live underground, because not wearing that 'happy face' is offensive to a subjugator culture that won't examine its own flaws. Do you fear the painful process of change? Why do you think you are exempt from change, when all around you, all other creatures and plants on Earth, have had to adapt to the rigid grid you allow them to occupy?

Can we prise the Minotaur's disguise away from our shoulders? Tear our masks off and look at the world with a compassionate eye? How different things could be if we admit we are all suffering.

If the labyrinth was a woman, it would be an emotive galaxy of energy. A ventura wave journeying to source. A cold, green eye performing an autopsy. A shaman walking us to the heart so we can process the dark truth and find out what happened to us. When we walk, hand-in-hand, back to our lives on the outside, undulating waves and tides will be powerful antidotes to hostile places. We cannot process the source of our agony when we are numbed with pharmaceuticals and trapped by amnesia and toxic tentacles. We must seek refuge in wild, natural places.

What if pain is a portal to the Otherworld? A tunnel of forgotten dreams. A doorway to the spirits. Somewhere to sit and meditate and absorb our story. What if pain became a sensation we can move through, where the edges are blurred? The freshwater swimming hole that we are desperate to get to.

What would you think if I told you that an underground spring has carved a cavern in the Limestone cliffs and that the walls of this natural labyrinth are like a gallery? It is a mineral temple, a shrine to abundance, honoured by millennia of humanity and the rippling walls sparkle with layers of crystal. Dynamic images, drawn with anatomical precision by ancient cave woman artists, describe a lush vision of a land of milk and honey. Herds of horses, panthers, bison and rhinoceros gallop across the walls of the glittering quartz passageways as if they were drawn yesterday.

Would you believe me if I told you that a Minotaur inhabits this cave? Half woman, half bison, she is 30,000 years old. A shaman, a healer who can blur the edges, communicate with the animal spirits, talk with Mother Earth and access the knowledge of sentient water and crystal, the keepers of memory. When she returns from her mystical trance, she can tell us about the Akashic Record, the Siren's sigh, a cosmic library of universal history, where every spoken word, intention and emotion is stored, stretching from the past, into the future. She can help us recall and process our story, rewire our neurons and rediscover the divine within. The voice of the Siren will return to us and when we reclaim our story it'll be our body's own wisdom that will heal us.

When we heal, we will see that man waged war on the mother who gave birth to him, because he misses and yearns for the nurture that only a matriarchal society can give him. He is lost. Man has created a dominator system that traumatises its sons because they can only do what the system requires them to do WHEN THEY FEEL NOTHING.

If pain is a labyrinth
Let me be your shaman
We can walk the left-hand spiral
Then take the right
Because the story of how we were wounded
Is best not faced alone

# *Kali II*

## Michelle Moirai

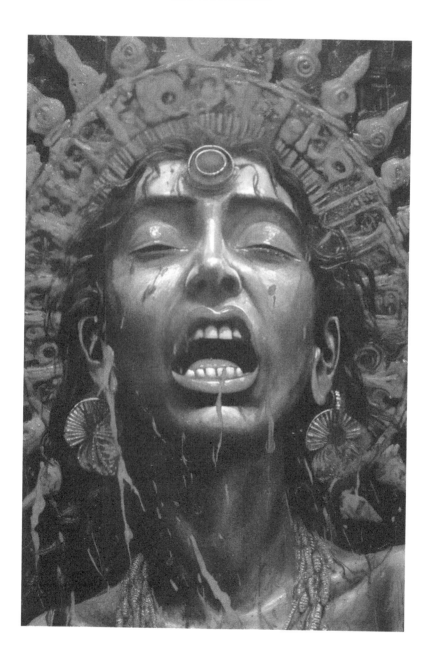

# You Know This Now

### Rebekah Myers

You may be suffering.
You may be deep in sorrow.
You may be truly alone and afraid.
Let the waves of anguish come.
Let them sweep over and through you.
Breathe.
Deep, slow breaths.
Hold on to the idea of love as you meet
the nightmare in the dark.
Hold on.
You may still be there when morning comes again.
The fever can break, and in the cool wafting winds of dawn, relief
may come to you.
You may hear birdsong, clear and sweet.
You may be visited by those beyond the veil.
Their love may feel like liquid golden light pouring down upon you.
Joy may come to you in simple, small ways—joy you thought you
might never know again—and when it does, learn to recognize it
for what it is.
Serendipity.
A gift not sought for.

And from this, let a knowledge be surely born in you.
You can pass through pain.
You can come out on the other side.
Joy is as real as sorrow.
And though this cycle may repeat itself throughout your lifetime,
you have learned to navigate the dangerous day.
You have learned to integrate your own devastation.

You have learned that you will always emerge,
in one way or another.
You will always be reborn.
Suffering will always be transformed.
Joy will always await you.
You know this now.


Rebekah Myers, Copyright 6/30/2021

# Women of Eriu

Barbara O'Meara

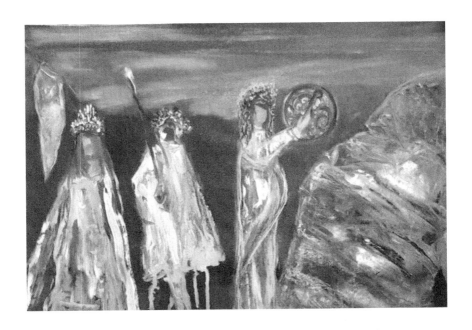

# Feeling the Pain

## Trista Hendren

As we were wrapping up this anthology, I received a surprising message letting me know that my beloved sister and long-time Girl God contributor, Barbara O'Meara, was in the final stages of dying. She thought she was in remission. The week that followed was excruciating knowing my beloved friend was in so much pain.

As is often the case, I turned to one of my favorite books for comfort: *The Great Cosmic Mother.*

> "If God is the Mother of the Universe, then the Creation is of the same substance as her—it is of her, as the child is of its mother's substance, and this means that the whole Creation is divine, and divinely related.
>
> We should have imagined life as created in the birth pain of God the Mother, then we would understand that—we would know that—our life's rhythm beats from Her great heart torn with agony of love and birth... Then we should understand why we Her children have inherited pain and we would feel that death meant a reunion with Her, a passing back into Her substance... the blood of Her blood again... Peace of Her Peace."[14]

I wish I had read these words as a young girl. I wish all children grew up reading this book instead of the patriarchal texts. We would live in an entirely different universe.

Pain has been a lifetime companion.

---

[14] Sjöö, Monica and Mor, Barbara. *The Great Cosmic Mother: Rediscovering the Religion of the Earth.* HarperOne; 2nd edition, 1987.

As a child, I used to wish I would get cancer so I would die. I'm sure this later translated into chronic pain.

I have suffered from migraines and constant back pain since my late teens. For the most part, I have learned to manage my symptoms. My migraines went away after leaving an abusive marriage and setting forth on a new path. My back pain is no longer a daily infliction. I have had to retrain my body out of my pain condition with radical self-care. I realize that this is not possible for many women on this planet. However, it is my vision for all of us. We can start, like I did, a little at a time, incorporating what we can afford financially and time-wise.

I do not believe any of us are meant to live with constant suffering. While illness and death are inevitable for all of us at some point, I believe we are meant to live with joy.

Pain still shows up for me when I am triggered or in a stressful situation. My back pain will revert to the same intensity when I am grieving, worrying, or out of balance. The regular practices of grounding, using tuning forks, fire cupping, deep stretching and self-massage are necessities for my well-being. I suspect as much for most of us with extensive trauma.

I came to feminism in college—before really immersing myself in Goddess Spirituality. I often say that Andrea Dworkin's words are, unfortunately, timeless.

> "One of the things the women's movement does is to make you feel pain. You feel your own pain, the pain of other women, the pain of sisters whose lives you can barely imagine. You have to have a lot of courage to accept that if you commit yourself, over the long term, not just for three months, not for a year, not for two years, but for a lifetime, to feminism, to the women's movement, that you are going to live with a lot of pain. In this country that is not a fashionable thing to do. So be prepared for the therapists.

And be prepared for the prescriptions. Be prepared for all the people who tell you that it's your problem, it's not a social problem, and why are you so bitter, and what's wrong with you? And underneath that is always the presumption that the rape was delusional, that the battery did not happen, that the economic hardship is your own unfortunate personal failing. Hold onto the fact that that's not true: it has never been true."[15]

Understanding the systematic oppressions that constitute patriarchy is a game-changer. It can also be very bleak. Women need each other. I fear now, more than ever we are becoming increasingly fragmented. That has been a frequent tactic used by patriarchs since male-centered monotheism took over.

Sitting in circles and sharing our stories is deeply healing. It is time for us to re-imagine a world we want to live in – where we can all thrive. As Diane Stein wrote:

> "Central to Women's Spirituality is the concept of women's self-empowerment, and this is central in women's Goddess rituals. Rituals in Women's spirituality create a microcosm, a 'little universe' within which women try out what they want the macrocosm, the 'big universe' or the real world to be."[16]

A few days after Barbara passed, war broke out again in the Middle East. Early one morning, feeling utterly devastated, I called in all the Foremother's I could think of who had passed... and then all the Goddesses. I asked them for direction, but heard no answer.

---

[15] Dworkin, Andrea. "Feminism: An Agenda," *Letters from a War Zone (1976-1989)*. Dutton; 1989.

[16] Stein, Diane from the Introduction to *The Goddess Celebrates: an Anthology of Women's Rituals*, Edited by Diane Stein. The Crossing Press; 1991.

I waited in the silence.

I began to feel the most intense pain and sadness. And then I wept.

I believe this was their answer. We have to feel the pain. And then we have to act.

We have at least 5,000 years of pain and grief built up in our collective DNA. The act of healing ourselves individually will shake loose the grip of patriarchal oppression. When enough of us heal, it will create a title wave: War and oppression will cease.

May the warm embrace of Her Peace bring comfort and healing to the entire world.

# List of Contributors

**Alison Newvine** is psychotherapist, singer/songwriter and a nature-loving, queer creative. Her psychotherapy and consultation practice centers around trauma healing, archetypal and spiritual inquiry and empowerment work with women, gender expansive folks, couples and the queer community. Along with her band, Spiral Muse, she writes and produces music dedicated to the Divine Feminine. Her band is currently recording their third original album, "Fire of Hope," centering around themes of rebirth and healing, set for release this winter. She is also developing songs for an Underworld Goddess album. She and her spouse live in the Bay Area, California with their beautiful black cat, Luz.

**Arna Baartz** is a painter, writer/poet, martial artist, educator and mother to eight fantastic children. She has been expressing herself creatively for more than 40 years and finds it to be her favourite way of exploring her inner being enough to evolve positively in an externally focused world. Arna's artistic and literary expression is her creative perspective of the stories she observes playing out around her. Claims to fame: Arna has been selected for major art prizes and won a number of awards, published many books, and— (her favourite) was used as a 'paintbrush' at the age of two by well-known Australian artist John Olsen. Arna lives and works from her bush studio in the Northern Rivers, NSW Australia. Her website is: www.artofkundalini.com

**Barbara O'Meara** (April 11th, 1963 – October 5th, 2023) was a professional visual artist, art activist, published writer & co-editor of *Soul Seers Irish Anthology of Celtic Shamanism*. Her 20 Solo Exhibitions included 'B.O.R.N.Babies of Ravaged Nations'. International juried shows include ASWM 'Wisdom Across the Ages', Lockhart Gallery New York 'Contemporary Irish Art' & Herstory 'Brigid's of the World' & 'Black Lives Matter'. Community Arts include 'Stitched With Love' Tuam Baby Blanket laid out onsite at the Mother & Child Institution by survivors and families, at KOLO International Women's Non Killing Cross Borders Summit in Sarajevo and held by Bosnian women war survivors. 'Sort Our Smears' Campaign at 'Festival of FeminismS'. 'Home Words Bound' publication with National Collective of Community Based Women's Networks where her paintings accompany writing by Irish women about the Pandemic. She continually developed empowering women's 'Art as Activism' projects through her final weeks. She was honoured to feature in many Girl God Books including as featured artist of *My Name is Brigid,* which launched on Brigid's Day 2022.

Barbara passed peacefully in the care of her beloved family on October 5th, 2023. She was in the midst of compiling *Sacred Breasts: an Inspirational Anthology for Living Your Breast Life.* The anthology will be completed and published in her honor by her co-editors. Her longtime sister-friend Dr. Karen Ward stepped up in her place to join the editing team. An anthology about Brigid is also in the works, dedicated to her memory and vision. www.barbaraomearaartist.com

**Betsy Long** grew up in Rome NY, and is now living in Socorro, New Mexico. She has lived all over the Rocky Mountains in the last 30 years. She recently married her high school love after being divorced from an 18-year marriage that wasn't right for her. She is a self-taught artist, with 4 children (2 of her, 2 from her husband), and 3 grandchildren, one of which she is planning a Red Tent ritual for soon.

**Claire Dorey**

Goldsmiths: BA Hons Fine Art.

Main Employment: Journalist and Creative, UK and overseas.

Artist: Most notable group show; Pillow Talk at the Tate Modern. Included in the Pillow Talk Book.

Curator: 3 x grass roots SLWA exhibitions and educational events on the subject of Female Empowerment, showcasing female artists, academic speeches and local musicians. Silence Is Over – Raising awareness on violence towards women; Ex Voto –

Existential Mexican Art Therapy; Heo – Female empowerment in the self- portrait.

Extra study: Suppressed Female History: History of the Goddess; Accessing Creative Wisdom; Sound and Breath Work; Reiki Master; Colour Therapy; Hand Mudras; Reflexology; Sculpture. Teaching Workshops: Sculpture and Drawing.

**Deborah A. Meyerriecks** is a retired NYC*EMS Lieutenant, Witch, and Community Priestess for over 20 years. She now resides in the liminal space between river, mountain, and desert in the Northwest of Arizona. A contributing author for Girl God Books since first submitting her essay, *Finding the Strength to Love Again for Warrior Queen* in early 2020. She now appears in 9 Girl God Book anthologies. Deborah's first book, *Macha and the Medic* was published on her birthday in 2021. She co-authored *Living In Magick* while continuing to work on her next books. Her work as priestess led her to the creation of the Shadow Care Retreats where she is honored to facilitate others with their personal Shadow Dive and Shadow Work, holding space for them, while lifting a lantern in the darkness to help others find their way back to themselves. Connect with her at: www.WillowMoonConsulting.com

**Geo Bitgood** is a holistic psychotherapist in the Pacific Northwest helping women recover from complex trauma, patriarchy stress, body battles, anxiety, and depression. She finds joy via dancing, nature adventures, and watching corgis be corgis.

**Kohenet Dr. Harriette E. Wimms** is a Maryland licensed clinical psychologist who provides compassion-infused mental health care to children, adolescents, adults, and families. Kohenet Wimms is a prayer leader in both the Kohenet community and Hinenu: The Baltimore Justice Shtiebl. She is the driving force behind Hinenu JOC, the Baltimore JOC Community Havurah, the Jews of Color Mishpacha Project. Harriette is currently a Keshet contract trainer, a Kesher mentor, and a member of the Seleh Jewish Leadership

Fellowship program, JOC cohort 17. A community connector, Kohenet Dr. Wimms is a proud, Fat, Disabled, Queer, Black, Jew by Choice, and is most proud of being mother to her 18-year-old son.

**Jeanine Elizabeth Otte** is a writer, poet, educator, and social change co-creator. Jeanine inspires a radical shift in thinking and living by uncovering the ancient wisdom of Earth and ordinary people, and sharing her visions for a caring, whole world. Jeanine creates at the intersection of the environment, economy, race, gender, family, body autonomy, and experiences of women and children. Jeanine is a certified conversation leader for a caring economy through the Center for Partnership Systems, a member of the Community Advisory Council for the Chicago Children's Advocacy Center, and inaugural alumna of the Quentin D. Young Equity Project connecting practitioners of social equity across sectors. She is a partner to Carlos and parent to Malcolm, Michelle, and Nicole.

**Kat Shaw** prides herself on breaking through the stereotypical views of beauty that have been cast upon society by the media, having made her name painting the glorious reality that is a woman's body. Her nude studies of real women garnered unprecedented popularity within only a few short months, as women were crying out for themselves to be portrayed in art, rather than the airbrushed images of the perfect female form that are so rife in today's culture.

After graduating with a fine art degree, Kat achieved a successful full-time teaching career for 14 years, and continues to teach art part-time whilst passionately pursuing her mission of world domination by empowering as many women as possible to reach their fullest potential by embracing their bodies and loving themselves wholeheartedly. Kat spreads her inspirational magic through her artwork, her Wellbeing business "Fabulously Imperfect", and her dedication to Goddess energy.

Reiki is a huge part of her life, and as a Reiki Master, Kat is committed to sharing Reiki, teaching Usui, Angelic and Karuna

Reiki, and channelling Reiki energy through her artwork to uplift and heal.

As a Sister of Avalon, Kat also works directly with her Goddess consciousness, connecting to Goddess and Priestess energy and translating it into Divine Feminine infused paintings to inspire women and spread Goddess love.

Kat is also mum to a gorgeous teenage daughter, a bellydancer and an avid pioneer to improve the lives of rescue animals.

**Kay Louise Aldred** is a researcher, writer, and educator, who catalyses individual, institutional and collective evolution – through education, embodiment, and creativity – amalgamating metacognition, intuition, and instinct.

She has published three workbooks of her own with Girl God Books – *Mentorship of Goddess: Growing Sacred Womanhood, Making Love with the Divine: Sacred, Ecstatic, Erotic Experiences* and *Somatic Shamanism: Your Fleshy Knowing as the Tree of Life* – in addition to co-authoring *Embodied Education: Creating Safe Space for Learning Facilitating and Sharing* with her husband Dan Aldred. The couple reside in North Yorkshire, England. www.kaylouisealdred.com, Instagram, Twitter and LinkedIn @kaylouisealdred

**Laura Valenti** is a qualified Movement Medicine teacher, a somatic and trauma-informed coach, a somatic stress release practitioner, and a holistic voice therapist.

Her profound curiosity and love for learning have propelled her on a two-decade-long journey of studying various spiritual philosophies and healing arts.

Laura's diverse background spans law, sociology of migration, physical theatre, clowning, and human rights advocacy. Her passion led her to travel internationally, and she has shared her skills with indigenous communities, individuals in drug and alcohol rehabilitation, refugees, women who have survived domestic violence, and vulnerable children.

She's a Moon dancer, a nomad at heart, profoundly cherishing community, music, drums, wilderness, and ceremony. Her roots trace back to Italy, where she learned the art of good food, the warmth of hospitality, and the vibrant nuances of colourful language.

Laura is currently embarking on a new adventure to become a Somatic Experience practitioner, adding to her repertoire of healing modalities. She views this as the next step in her dedication to the community's well-being and healing intergenerational trauma.

Her journey took an unexpected turn when chemotherapy induced premature menopause. Rather than resisting this change, she embraced it as an initiation and rite of passage, firmly believing in the pivotal role of older women as wisdom keepers.

For a deeper dive into Laura's transformative work, please visit her website: www.elementalsoulmedicine.com

**Lucy H. Pearce** is driven by a need to create, connect and inspire. A best-selling author, vibrant artist, respected publisher and editor. Often described as raw, authentic and life-changing, her work encourages authentic paths to self-expression and is celebrated particularly by highly sensitive and neurodivergent women.

Her award-winning books include: *Burning Woman; Creatrix; Moon Time; Medicine Woman; She of the Sea; Crow Moon; Full Circle Health; The Rainbow Way.*

Lucy is the founder and creative director of Womancraft Publishing, established in 2014, which publishes life-changing, paradigm-shifting books by women, for women. She is the mother of three and lives on the south coast of Ireland. Contact her here:
www.lucyhpearce.com
www.womancraftpublishing.com

**Michelle Moirai** is a digital artist who lives and works in Morgantown, West Virginia. Her personal style focuses on duplication of traditional art mediums in a digital setting, and the themes of transformation and uncovering what has been hidden.

Currently, Moirai works as the Assistant Director of Marketing Technology for the Benjamin M. Statler College of Engineering and Mineral Resources at West Virginia University, where she uses her design talents to create websites for the college. Outside of work, she continues to create digital paintings, and is currently exploring how text-to-art artificial intelligence can be beneficial to the advancement of the digital arts.
https://mementomoirai.com/

**Pat Daly** (editor) is a mother of three daughters and proud grandma. A published author / writer on career and job search issues, Pat is semi-retired and lives in Portland, Oregon.

**Rachael Noton** is a figurative artist, focusing on the empowerment of the woman's body. Having always loved colour in her art, she uses it in such a way that is abstract and flowing, just as the woman's body is, free flowing – and like a woman-dances. Rachael started off by intuitively painting and drawing, but now that she has been to college she uses her skills and knowledge as well as her intuition. Rachael feels drawn to spiritual art and loves the feeling of the unknown, so when she puts brush to canvas she is pulled in a direction that just isn't known yet, and her art is born.

**Siobhan Finnegan** lives in London. She originally trained as a contemporary dancer and then a fitness instructor, before becoming an Occupational Therapist in her late twenties. These work experiences along with general life events generated a number of questions, such as 'what are we actually doing here? 'and 'why are we doing it like this?'. These questions either went unanswered or the responses were unsatisfactory. Siobhan experienced the consequences of being silenced as a traumatic process and is aware that this is not an uncommon experience for those who question institutions.

During this time Siobhan was also dealing with her own physical pain, which failed to be taken seriously by a number of health practitioners. She intends to write about these experiences and is interested in creating work to explore other women's experiences of having their pain dismissed by health professionals.

Her experiences prompted a return to study and she undertook a masters in Gender, Media and Culture at Goldsmiths University London. This enabled her to explore feminist and post-colonial theory and create papers that looked at embodiment and the social constructs of identities, including those of the patient-doctor dynamic. To explore the colonial ghosts that still haunt medical systems and to produce a dissertation that positioned trauma in the culture rather than existing merely as individual issues. This piece also looked at the broader medical cultures which enables poor practice to flourish unnoticed, due to power dynamics, vested interests and bias belief systems about bodies, in particular the bodies of women.

Siobhan would be keen to hear from others interested in this area, through lived experience or otherwise. She can be contacted on Siobhanfinnegan3@gmail.com.

**Rev Sionainn McLean** is a polytheist fire witch and animist, on a crazy spiritual journey over the last 25 years. She believes that our spiritual path is always growing and evolving, moving in a spiral as we explore what moves our higher self. She is a priestess of The Morrigan and has served the Great Queen for over 5 years. She is a graduate of both the Community Ministry program and the Spiritual Direction Program with Cherry Hill Seminary, and ordained with Sacred Wells Congregation. She is the owner and operator of Liminal Raven Ministries whose mission is to aid in self-empowerment, provide inspiration, guidance, support and ministry to pagans as well as to nurture spiritual growth in others. She serves as a spiritual companion and priest. She's also a mom, wife, writer, painter and gardener.

**Dr. Stephanie Mines** is the author of five books that reflect over three decades of research as a neuroscientist. She has investigated shock and trauma as a survivor, a professional, a clinical researcher, and healthcare provider. Her nonprofit The TARA Approach is instrumental in the systemic change she promotes as a Regenerative Health paradigm.

Dr. Mines also developed Climate Change & Consciousness to facilitate inner transformation for grounded climate action. Climate Change & Consciousness serves an international and intergenerational community of visionary activists.

In addition, Dr. Mines is an award-winning poet. Her poetry has been published in anthologies and in chapbooks.

Dr. Mines' latest book, *Memoir of An Embryologist: How I Discovered the Secret of Resilience*, was released in 2023 from Inner Traditions/Sacred Planet Books.

**Sylvia Rose** is a retired social worker and a long-time witch in the Reclaiming tradition. She has had ME for nearly half her life and is currently severely affected – which gives her plenty of time these days to lie in bed thinking, reading and writing.

**Tamara Albanna** has always been connected to the Goddess, even when she didn't realize it. As a Doula and Childbirth Educator, she witnessed divinity first-hand through other women. Now as a writer, artist, Reiki healer and Tarot reader, she hopes to help others overcome their difficult pasts while healing with the Divine Mother. She has published two books on Inanna—*Inanna's Ascent: Reclaiming Female Power* (co-edited with Trista Hendren and Pat Daly) and *My Name is Inanna*; two books on Willendorf—*Willendorf's Legacy: The Sacred Body* (co-edited with Trista Hendren and Pat Daly) and *My Name is Goddess of Willendorf*—as well as three poetry chapbooks, *As I Lay By the Tigris and Weep, Rosewater, Kismet* and *Kissing the Moon*. Tamara currently resides in Europe with her family. Website: https://tamara-albanna.com.

**Traci Purwin** creatively expresses her Neurodiversity in as many mediums as possible. She has adopted Ireland as her homeland and lives by the sea in Cork with her family. www.tracipurwin.com

**Trista Hendren** founded Girl God Books in 2011 to support a necessary unraveling of the patriarchal world view of divinity. Her first book—*The Girl God*, a children's picture book—was a response to her own daughter's inability to see herself reflected in God. Since then, she has published more than 50 books by a dozen women from across the globe with help from her family and friends. She lives in Bergen, Norway. You can learn more about her projects here: www.thegirlgod.com

**Victoria Earle** is a freelance writer and Features Editor of the sustainable lifestyle magazine *Frank* (thefrankmagazine.com). She has also trained as a Soul Healer with the Glastonbury Goddess Temple. She is working on her own healing and unbinding herself from patriarchy and internalised misogyny.

**Victoria Louise Lapping** has a lifelong passion for Storytelling and has gained Masters of the Arts in Film Production to further this passion.

She loves how the art of Storytelling can help with life experiences, especially as she is someone who fits outside current social constructs with being chronically disabled and identifying as gay.

Victoria has a diverse range of experiences and qualifications from a background in Musical Theatre, Film and TV, and training in a wide range of areas, including Astrology.

Her family-owned holistic shop (Crystal Moon Emporium) birthed a lifelong passion for spiritualty, working with Goddesses, Crystals and Mother Earth. They have taught her Druidry, witchcraft, paganism, and shamanism among many other paths.

In addition, she is undertaking Priestess training in Astrology and Morgan LeFay. She is very grateful to get to live her dream and live her life calling as a Writer.

# Trista's Acknowledgments

I would like to acknowledge my co-editors. My mother, **Pat Daly,** has edited each and every one of my books. There would be no Girl God Books without her enormous contributions. I was thrilled to also work with **Kay Louise Aldred** on this project as well—who fast became a sister.

Tremendous gratitude to **Kat Shaw** for allowing us to feature her gorgeous painting as the cover art.

Enormous appreciation to my husband **Anders Løberg**, who prepared the document for printing and helped with website updates. Your love, support and many contributions made this book possible.

Lastly, I would like to thank my dear sisters **Tamara Albanna, Susan Morgaine, Jeanette Bjørnsen, Camilla Berge Wolff, Sharon Smith, Arlene Bailey, Barbara O'Meara, Tammy Nedrebø-Skurtveit, Kay Louise Aldred, Kat Shaw, Arna Baartz** and **Alyscia Cunningham** for always being right there to cheer me on in the spirit of true sisterhood.

Thank you to all our readers and Girl God supporters over the years. We love and appreciate you!

## Kay's Acknowledgments

I'd like to thank all the women have shared so authentically and offered such powerful art and writing this book.

Gratitude to **Trista Hendren** for founding Girl God Books and her ongoing commitment to women, and Goddess. Thank you for cocreating with me and your yes.

Huge appreciation to my co-editor **Pat Daly** and to **Kat Shaw** for the inspiring cover art.

Thank you to all of those who been a companion when I was in pain. Thank you for staying. Thank you for your soothing, loving, presence.

And finally huge love and appreciation for my husband **Dan** and his endless encouragement and engagement with pain, pleasure and passion.

**If you enjoyed this book, please consider writing a brief review on Amazon and/or Goodreads.**

# What's Next?!

*Kali Rising: Holy Rage* – Edited by C. Ara Campbell, Jaclyn Cherie, Trista Hendren and Pat Daly

*Wounded Feminine: Grieving with Goddess* – Edited by Claire Dorey, Trista Hendren, and Pat Daly

*Sacred Breasts: an Inspirational Anthology for Living Your Breast Life* – Edited by Barbara O'Meara, Dr. Karen Ward, Trista Hendren and Pat Daly

*Goddess Chants and Songs Book* – Edited by Trista Hendren and Pat Daly

*And Still, I Rise* – Kat Shaw

http://thegirlgod.com/publishing.php

Made in the USA
Middletown, DE
06 November 2023